SLIMMER AND HEALTHIER

CREATING A SLIM, HEALTHY BODY FOR LIFE

BY DEBORAH BROMLEY
IN COLLABORATION WITH HEMI-SYNC®

FEATURING A BIOGRAPHY OF ROBERT MONROE

Written by Deborah Bromley 2019
Published by Flying Man Books™ 2019
Interstate Industries, Inc. dba Flying Man Books™
P.O. Box 505, Lovingston
VA 22949
https://hemi-sync.com

ISBN: 978 1 712 476024

The information contained in this book is provided as supporting guidance to the Hemi-Sync® album of verbally-guided meditations of the same name. The information is not intended to be relied upon as constituting medical advice. Readers should always consult an appropriate medical professional prior to making changes to their diet and lifestyle which may impact on their health. The author and publisher specifically disclaim any liability, loss or risk, either personal or otherwise, that is incurred as a direct or indirect consequence of the use or application of any of the contents of this book.

The 12 verbally-guided meditations in the album are accompanied by Hemi-Sync® music and audio tones which support the verbal guidance. Hemi-Sync® is a safe, time-proven technology. However, if you have a tendency towards seizures, auditory disorders or adverse mental conditions, do not listen to Hemi-Sync® without first consulting your physician. In the unlikely event you experience any physical or mental discomfort, immediately discontinue use. While many of Hemi-Sync® products contribute to wellness, they are not intended to replace medical diagnosis and treatment. All warranties whether express or implied, including warranties of merchantability and fitness for a particular purpose, are disclaimed. Do not listen to Hemi-Sync® products while driving.

CONTENTS

INTRODUCTION

This book accompanies the Hemi-Sync® album, *Slimmer and Healthier — Creating a Slim, Healthy Body for Life*. Taken together, the guided meditations and the supporting information in this book have been designed to be exactly like a course of therapy sessions, personalized to fit your requirements. This program can all be experienced in the comfort of your own home, at your own pace, learning as you go. You will discover things about yourself and fine-tune your progress to fit your life circumstances and the goals you are aiming for.

Slimmer and Healthier is a program for those who wish to make changes in their life regarding their weight, body image, their nutrition and their health. Enjoying good health is not dependent on what size or shape you are, it is more complex than that. However, when you use this program you will learn how to listen to what you body wants in terms of your nutrition, your lifestyle, your wellbeing and sense of self. Guided meditations may promote positive mental and emotional changes, including the reduction of stress in your life. There are many benefits for health and wellbeing. These ideas will be explored in more detail in the guided meditations and in this book.

The audio program consists of 12 verbally-guided meditations carefully planned to encompass all aspects of a successful weight loss program. With the addition of the explanations, examples and background information in this companion book, you will discover deep inner truths about yourself, including the ways your mind and emotions influence your eating and your weight. You'll find out how to let go of everything that is holding you back. You will build the positive mindset that ensures success.

Becoming slimmer and healthier can be a celebration of the joy of inhabiting your body with all of your being. It is an *inner* process, involving your body, mind, emotions and "life force" energy. A journey of weight loss that transforms you in this way cannot be separated from your day-to-day life. It's possible that your weight and body image are having a profound effect on who you are, how you feel about yourself and how you live your life. Therefore, this program will address, in a positive and healing way, all aspects of your life that you may want to change.

You may already recognize that what is happening in your life has direct links to your body weight and shape. You might understand that serious change is needed. This program is designed to support those changes in a way that is both gentle and healing, but tough and effective. You want to create your slim, healthy body for life. You want results. This program begins with the clear priority of getting the process of becoming slimmer and healthier started. During the journey, you will develop positive changes to your everyday habits, your thinking, your emotions and your zest for living, integrated into the deepest part of you.

It doesn't matter where you begin. It doesn't matter how many times you have tried, struggled and given up. It doesn't matter how many challenges there are in your life situation, your health, your schedule or your abilities. Everyone who wishes to create a slimmer, healthier body for life will benefit from this program. It works on the *causes* of unwanted weight, rather than being limited to the *symptoms*. All the time, you will be in control of what goals you want to aim for. That is because the only person who can make these decision is *you*.

There are no recipes or food plans in this program. This is a deliberate omission. At the heart of successful weight loss is the truth that your personal tastes, preferences and lifestyle should dictate what you eat. Enjoyment must be at the center of your meal times. If you normally try to lose weight with a diet that is strict and punishing, eating food that makes you feel unwell and unhappy, you may experience doubts about this idea. Surely it's impossible to achieve a slim, healthy body by enjoying yourself?

Actually, the *exact opposite* is true. When you enjoy what you are doing, you naturally want to do more of it. It will therefore be easy to keep going. Before long, eating this way will become effortless and automatic. After a month or two, you will not have to put any thought or energy into eating less but enjoying it more. You will continue to lose weight. This will be a complete reversal of what you are accustomed to. If your past experience of diets is clouded with memories of hunger, unpleasant food, strict regimes and, ultimately, of giving up, you are in for a lovely surprise.

Think about the diet plans you have tried in the past. There are so many to choose from, all weird and wonderful, all promising successful weight loss as long as you follow the program exactly. At the heart of most diet programs is restriction. What you can and can't have. What you must and must not do. What foods and drinks you must give up. What strange and unpleasant meals you have to eat to lose weight. As if you should to be punished for being overweight in the first place. Incidentally, if any of these diets worked and were successful, I doubt you'd be reading this book.

Simply expressed, the best diet for you is the one that includes all the foods you love to eat in *just the right amounts*. Your body, mind and emotions have an important role to play in deciding what you love to eat. How foods make you feel physically, mentally and emotionally will define what these foods are. There are no right or wrong foods. Only what is right or wrong for you. It is not up to me or any scientist or doctor or nutritionist or government advisory body to tell you what foods you love to eat, give you pleasure and make you feel good inside.

However, when you truly listen to your body you may be surprised at what it is telling you. Be prepared to learn what your body, mind and emotions actually want you to eat. When you really taste your food, every mouthful, every flavor, every texture, that's when you can decide what you love to eat.

Think of it like this. You already have all the equipment — very sophisticated equipment — inside your body to make the right choices about what foods are good for you. Your eyes, nose, lips and tongue are fully set up to help you. Your mind remembers what foods made you feel good, not just while you ate them but also during the hours afterwards. Your stomach has sophisticated sensors to register hunger and fullness. Your body monitors blood sugar, checking that you have enough energy for your activity levels. Your skin, your hair, your smile and the sparkle in your eyes all register the quality of the nourishment in the food you eat. You are an individual, with likes and dislikes, foods that upset your balance or make you feel unwell. That is why it's vital to listen to your body, mind and emotions and take notice of the messages about what foods are right for you.

You will learn everything you need to know in this book and by using the Hemi-Sync® album in the prescribed way. It has been made deliberately enjoyable for you. You will feel better inside from the start by following this program because it is positive, life-enhancing and interesting. It will be like an adventure. There are extra benefits from using verbally-guided meditation in this way. You will reduce stress in your life. You'll learn how to relax your mind and let go of things that bother you. You'll grow in confidence. These simple and natural extra benefits from this program will also be important to your weight loss. For example:

- Stress tends to result in the body storing fat rather than releasing energy for you to use. Stress hormones are at the root of this process and they can have a significant negative impact on your ability to lose weight.
- When you are tense and anxious or can't slow your mind down, you are more likely to turn to food or alcohol to help you relax and unwind.
- If you lack confidence in your own ability to follow a weight loss program, doubts can creep in and increase the probability that you give up.

More explanation about how each of the guided meditations work and how to get the best out of each track can be found in the 12 chapters in this book, each one relating to a specific track.

There are no negative messages in this program, no aversion therapy or suggestions to cut out "bad" foods. There is no place for negativity on this journey towards being slimmer and healthier. I suspect you already have a whole truckload of unhelpful, self-defeating thoughts, ideas and beliefs on the subject of your weight. The objective of this program is to heal and dissolve all of that negativity while allowing you to create your slim, healthy body for life. All of this is possible. Decide now to give this program 100%. You won't regret it.

HOW TO USE THIS BOOK
The audio program is designed to be a complete package, containing everything you need to create a slim, healthy body for life. There are instructions about to how often you need to use each audio track

(some are core tracks, some are optional), how to get the best out of each track and what to expect. It's good, however, to be able to fill in some background details and understand how and why things work. It's interesting to find out how your mind, emotions and life force energy influence your weight. You will also learn more about the therapies that are utilized in this process. Being fully informed brings more power and energy to your weight loss journey.

If the audio program represents a full course of therapy sessions, this book is the incidental therapy chat that goes with it. Each audio track is explained in detail so you can satisfy yourself that you fully understand what you are doing and why you are doing it.

You can read each part of this book as you use the relevant audio track, ensuring that you have all the information you need on that particular stage of the process. If you are naturally curious, you can read the entire book all at once. There is no right or wrong way to do this. Many people prefer to understand everything in advance before they begin.

Your overall experience as you undertake this program will be enhanced by being fully informed. Think of this book as your personal coach, cheering you on as you progress through your journey, reminding you what to expect, which part to do next, what you can skip or what needs more of your time and attention.

Everything you might need is here. Let your journey begin.

SUMMARY OF THE PROGRAM

Each track has a particular purpose for your weight loss journey. Seven of the tracks are core tracks to be utilized by everyone. The remaining five fulfill more specific roles. Study the guidance for each individual track to find out how often to use each track, what to expect and how to optimize your inner work. Many of the tracks refer to your "wise inner self," your internal supporter or cheerleader, who has your best interests at heart. When you have this wise inner self on your side, you will be unstoppable.

TRACKS 1, 2 & 3
The first four weeks, or thereabouts, of your weight loss journey will involve listening to these three core tracks on a regular basis, perhaps every day for the first few weeks. You will know when you have done enough. By immersing yourself in this part of the program you begin to lose weight right away.

Track 1 works on completely changing the way you think and act towards food. Your eating habits will change, so that you eat much less food but enjoy it more. Losing weight should be and will be a process filled with pleasure. There are no food rules to follow. You eat the foods you love and the foods that love you back. Your food choices will evolve as you progress, as you listen to what your body wants you to eat. It's important for you to decide what your body needs, rather than some distant diet expert who knows nothing about you.

In Track 2 you practice the skill of eating less but enjoying it more "live" while you eat your meal. You begin to lose weight right away as you practice this way of eating. By fully engaging with the experience of eating your meal while in a state of focused awareness, your mind readily accepts the changes to your eating habits. Soon you will do this automatically, without having to think about it. Overeating will be a thing of the past.

Track 3, a short track, is all about developing iron willpower which will strengthen your resolve to lose all your excess weight. These three opening tracks will provide you with everything you need to lose weight from the start of the program. New eating habits, new thoughts, ideas, emotions and beliefs will carry you forward.

TRACKS 4, 5 & 6
These optional tracks which supplement your core work will be of benefit to those who wish to change their relationship with food forever. You learn how to banish food cravings using a powerful acu-tapping technique in Track 4. Food will cease to have power over you.

Track 5 is for those who suspect they have a sluggish metabolism and want to have more energy. You work on boosting your metabolism and improving energy levels using visualization and clear instructions to your subconscious mind.

Track 6 is an innovative guided meditation that works by changing your mental mindset from negative into positive. You listen to the track and absorb the powerful commands that instruct your sleeping mind to run a night-time clean-up program while you sleep. You learn how to use the command phrase — slim while you sleep — so you can run the program automatically.

TRACKS 7, 8 & 9
Track 7 is a core track, a guided meditation to remove all obstacles that may be stopping you from creating the slim, healthy body you wish for. At the end of the track you visualize your slim future and practice walking towards it. If the past has power over you, including uncomfortable memories of past dieting failures, then Track 8 will help you let go of any negative influences. The past with all its difficult memories can therefore be healed. Track 9 will banish destructive self-sabotaging behaviors and help to overcome feelings of failure which can undermine your self-confidence.

TRACKS 10, 11 & 12
Track 10, a walking meditation, encourages you to walk while you meditate and refresh the main points of the program to create your

slim, healthy body. Walking also reduces stress and makes you feel energized. Track 11 is a short track of affirmations which you use while awake, repeating the phrases to firm up your resolve. Track 12 completes the program and takes you forwards with perseverance into your slim, healthy future. You listen to this track, as required, to keep you on target.

*****

Everyone is different, with unique requirements from a weight loss program. As you progress and lose weight, you may encounter unexpected challenges that have the potential to frustrate your progress or make you want to give up. You will gain the support you need from the optional tracks in this program.

Losing weight and creating a slim, healthy body takes time and energy. Make up your mind to give this program 100% by using the tracks as instructed and as often as required. Your life will improve as you work through the tracks, learning everything required to make your life exactly as you wish to be. Look forward to being slim and healthy, filled with confidence and having a harmonious, loving and respectful relationship with food. Commit now to do this for yourself.

CHAPTER 1

CREATING A SLIM, HEALTHY BODY

(BY EATING LESS BUT ENJOYING IT MORE)

> "This journey will be an amazing adventure, a delicious voyage of discovery for you that leads to a slim, healthy body."
> — *Creating a Slim, Healthy Body*, Track 1

This simple principle of losing weight is the foundation of the program. It sounds easy, too easy perhaps. It could be described as an *enjoyable challenge*. It's a way of eating that you learn to do, with all your outer senses and also with your deep inner knowing. Once you have this method of eating fully set in your mind, emotions and habits, eating this way soon becomes automatic. Little effort is required. You can focus completely on enjoying yourself as much as possible, both when you eat and when you are doing other things. And you can lose all your unwanted weight in the process.

Track 1 and Track 2 of the Hemi-Sync® program are devoted to eating less but enjoying it more. Track 1 is the core track, to be used regularly from the start of the program for several weeks. Track 2 is a waking version of the method, a guided meditation used while you are awake and practicing the skill of eating less but enjoying it more during your meal. By working at a deep level to absorb everything about this way of eating and then putting it into practice, you will be setting yourself up for success. The tracks, featuring Hemi-Sync® frequencies that will uniquely complement the verbal instructions, ensure these new habits are successfully taken deep into your subconscious.

You will be working primarily on this journey with your subconscious mind, but it's important to understand there is a role for your conscious mind to play. Paying attention to the waking element of this method (while you are eating your meals), and putting effort and energy into the process, will ensure complete success. Soon you will eat less but enjoy it more without having to consciously focus or think about what you are doing. You will do it automatically. Therefore, making this part of the process work is a priority. It must come first and be your primary focus until you are confident it is integrated into your subconscious, automatic behavior.

YOUR EATING HABITS WILL CHANGE
It is estimated it takes about 28 days for deeply embedded habits to change. Think about your current eating habits and how long they have been your default behavior. Do you eat breakfast on the go or in the car? Do you stand at the refrigerator nibbling at various foods while thinking about what to have for dinner? Do you finish up the children's leftovers because you don't like waste? Do you habitually watch TV when you eat? Or do you look at social media on your phone? Do you upsize when you choose a take-away meal? Do you always ditch your diet when you eat out?

Take a minute to think about your eating habits now. Be honest with yourself. And understand that these habits must change. It will take about 28 days to change them, and that will require a degree of per-sistence on your behalf. This is a short period of time compared to how long your current eating habits have been driving your behavior. The more effort you put in during this beginning phase, the better results you will get. And all the time you will be enjoying your food more than you have for a long time. I suggest that this time of effort and focus will seem like a wonderful adventure. Tell yourself it will be a hugely enjoy-able learning experience that will yield the most wonderful results.

Begin this process when you have a few days to relax and devote time to it. Behavior change doesn't really fit in well with a busy, high stress schedule. Make up your mind and choose a suitable time to start. Plan to have some quiet time, time that you can use to learn how to enjoy your food without any distractions.

For optimum results you will listen to Tracks 1 and 2 for about 28 days or as long as is needed to make sure your new eating habit is firmly set in your mind. You will know when this has occurred because you'll be eating less but enjoying it more without having to think about it. For extra variety in your meditations, Track 3 can be mixed into the first phase of your program and this will boost your willpower. Load these tracks onto a device flexible enough to use anytime, when you have a peaceful half-hour to do your inner work. Tell your family or those you live with that you do not want to be disturbed. Tell yourself it's your number one priority right now.

You may wonder what it will be like to practice meditation techniques in this way, and what you will experience. Common questions are, "How will I know I'm doing it right?" and "What does it feel like?" and "How will I know it's working?"

WHAT TO EXPECT FROM TRACKS 1 & 2
When you begin working with verbally-guided meditations, you may notice your mind struggles to settle down and relax. It may keep pitching in with other thoughts or distractions and that's okay. Keep bringing your focus back to the track. Become more involved with the words, images and music. Think of it as your special time for deep

relaxation, away from the pressures of your everyday life. Give yourself permission to put other thoughts to the side. You can pick them up when you've finished. As you practice, you'll notice how easy it becomes to focus more completely on the verbal guidance. The music leads you gently into deeper states of relaxation. This ability to slow your mind down and be more aware of the "now" is a skill that can be learned. Everyone can do it. It is inevitable that you will get better and better at it when you practice consistently. Your mind relaxes, you are able to focus moment by moment on what you are listening to. This an excellent skill to learn, because as you slow your mind down at your command, your ability to concentrate and focus all your attention on whatever you are doing will improve.

As you progress with your meditations and enjoy the mental relaxation, you may experience the sensation of your mind drifting. You may feel as if you missed some of the words, or you may think you've been asleep. Sensations of body dissociation may accompany this feeling, as if you are involved in a wonderful dream while you are awake. Congratulations! You are now experiencing altered states of awareness where your conscious mind slips out for a while, allowing your powerful subconscious mind to absorb the verbal guidance more fully.

There are many levels of altered and expanded states of awareness, all of them perfectly natural. You may find that some days your mind slips easily into these states and you only "wake up" when you get to the end of the track. Other days you may remain fully aware all the way through.

Be assured, your mind will always be listening and absorbing the instructions. The subconscious never sleeps. Enjoy what you are experiencing, use it for maximum benefit and learn as you go along. If you are one of those people who quickly goes into deep states, and are likely to drift off to sleep at the end of the track, you should set an alarm of some kind if you are listening during the day. While it's sometimes good to have a restorative nap, you don't want to sleep when you should be awake and getting on with your schedule. Be practical about this and do whatever is necessary.

TRACKS 1 & 2 WILL TOTALLY CHANGE YOUR EATING HABITS

You can use Track 1 at bedtime if you so choose. You may find yourself enjoying more relaxed sleep. I recommend, however, that optimum results come from also listening at other times during the day when your mind is more likely to take notice of the words and integrate them into both your conscious mind and subconscious mind.

Track 2 is for using when you are actually eating. Make your meal time experience more real by using this track to embed the powerful instructions and then link them in your mind to the eating-less-but-enjoying-it-more experience. This will be very beneficial when you start the process. Get competitive with yourself. Try out your favorite foods and find out exactly how much more you can enjoy them. Get up close to what "full" really means. Strengthen that link between your eyes, your nose, your mouth and your stomach. Make it real for yourself. But above all, have fun!

Maybe there are times in your day when you'd like to have something to listen to while you are taking the dog for a walk or doing the grocery shopping or clearing up the back yard. You can listen to the *Walking Meditation,* Track 10, with your eyes open. Your mind will adapt the "walking" instructions to whatever you are doing.

Track 11, *Affirmations for a Slim, Healthy Body,* are also useful and you do them in the waking state. Your mind is often drifting when you do tasks that are repetitive or habitual. Your subconscious mind will absorb the verbal guidance with no barriers in the way. *However, never, ever listen while doing anything that requires your full conscious attention to maintain safety.* Full mental concentration is required for any task that may result in harm to yourself or another person.

You may notice yourself thinking snippets of the words from the track as you go about your day. You may hear yourself say, "I am determined and focused on my goals," or "nothing is going to stop me." This is a sign your mind is enacting the guidance. You may just *sense* the powerful messages, and only notice when you do things differently. This is a very common experience. You suddenly become aware your habits have changed and you only realize it after the event.

However you experience the changes, it will be right for you. Go at your own pace but give it 100%. This is a long-term change process, not a quick fix. The changes will build up, they are cumulative and permanent. You will never go back to old ways of thinking, feeling and behaving, once you have successfully absorbed the verbal guidance and taken it deep inside you.

LETTING GO OF NEGATIVE FOOD ATTITUDES

There are many, many hidden benefits from learning to eat in this new way. The first and most important, apart from the weight loss, is the way this method has the potential to heal negative, toxic, unhelpful and damaging attitudes about food and eating. Many people have developed a complicated relationship with food. Food is something to be blamed, to feel guilty about, to be afraid of or to be angry about. Food is either good or bad. When you think about food in this way, you are either allowed to eat it or it's forbidden.

Such attitudes are easy to accumulate if you have been trying to lose weight for a while, and particularly if you read and absorb everything you read about in the media or online. It seems like every day brings a new scare about what foods are good or bad for your health, or new research that contradicts what you thought was true about foods you love. You might read about a strange sounding berry from a far-off country that you must now eat at every meal. Or perhaps you learn about a new fashionable juice that will cause all your unwanted weight to melt away and also cure all of humanity's illnesses.

When food takes over your mind in this way it can make you feel a bit crazy. I know that sounds dramatic, but when food obsession has you in its grip it feels like your mind is out of control. It is characterized by thinking about food from the moment you wake until the moment you go to sleep.

Another symptom of food obsession is when every calorie has to be counted, anguished over and judged. All your conversation revolves around food and your latest diet. It takes over your life. Nothing else matters except what you weigh and whether you are happy with that. Most likely you are not happy. This is no way to live and enjoy your life to the fullest. Therefore a great benefit of this way of eating is unraveling and releasing your obsession with food and eating and weight. It's good to have a harmonious and respectful relationship with food. This method will build that relationship. Food is meant to be a source of enjoyment. If it isn't, then it's time to let go of that way of thinking.

MATCHING YOUR DIET TO YOUR OWN LIKES AND DISLIKES

The best diet for you, the one that will be most successful, includes all the foods you enjoy and none of the foods you dislike. I sense the sound of disbelieving gasps. If you are a veteran of past weight loss campaigns, you will already have endured long days eating cabbage soup, weeks spent quitting sugar, dreary months eating only protein foods and long periods studying lots of different diet plans containing foods you can't pronounce and really, really don't like the taste of.

I have the T-shirt for this particular subject, and own all the bragging rights. No plan is so weird or unpleasant that I haven't tried it. I now hold firm to the logical conclusion that such plans are destined to fail. The simple truth is that people naturally have different likes and dislikes which creates a serious problem if you try to lose weight by sticking to a rigid eating plan. Within your family and circle of friends you'll know of the person who cannot abide mushrooms, or is allergic to seafood, or doesn't like the smell of garlic. You already know which foods you don't love and maybe the ones that *don't love you back*. Over time, you might notice that certain foods give you headaches, or make you feel sluggish or give you an upset stomach. It is so important to respect what your body is telling you. The majority of diet plans are based on inflexible rules that must be followed, no matter what. It is often claimed that following the diet exactly is the only way to lose weight. Right from the start you are faced with a food plan that includes foods and ways of eating that are alien to you.

The long term result of such diet plans is that you give up. When you switch from eating foods that you love and make you feel good, to a meal plan of strange food that has to be specially purchased and prepared, it might be exciting for a day or two, but after a few more days you begin to feel a bit lonely and fed up. You're eating different meals than everyone else. It's likely you won't be invited to join friends to go out to dinner. Nobody wants to listen to you talking about 20 tasty ways with spinach. You may feel isolated and a bit miserable. You definitely know you are on a diet. I'll bet you can't wait to give it up.

I wonder, what is the strangest diet you ever tried? Take a moment to remind yourself of all the things you had to do, the rules and do's and don'ts. Did you enjoy it? Were you successful?

When you base your meals on foods you already enjoy, you have the foundation for a good weight loss plan. This program fits with your schedule and your likes and dislikes. It respects the foods that don't agree with you. If you have a family, this eating plan already fits in with all the food preferences of everyone you care about. You will be able to continue making meals that everyone enjoys and this simple expedient makes transforming your own eating habits so much easier. Your budget also won't have to bear the strain of purchasing outlandish diet ingredients. You'll be able to concentrate on eating less but enjoying it more, rather than deciding how to make cakes out of vegetables. I love carrot cake, I cannot lie, but sometimes other vegetables need to know their place. If your zucchini muffins are your most prized recipe, I sincerely apologize and trust you'll continue to enjoy baking them and eating them.

LISTENING CAREFULLY TO YOUR BODY

Your body, mind and emotions are one system, balanced to perfection. When you really listen to what your body is telling you, you will surprise yourself with what you hear. Your body will send you signals about what it would really like you to eat. There are sensors everywhere inside checking for energy levels, protein requirements, fat usage, carbohydrate metabolism, vitamin levels and mineral concentrations. Your mind and emotions also add their input to help you decide what nourishment satisfies your needs at any particular moment.

Maybe you have already experienced this. You suddenly get the desire for a specific food. Or you are standing in front of the refrigerator looking at the contents when something draws your attention and you have to eat it right away.

It may seem to you that you *already* listen to what your body is telling you to eat. I answer back that you can listen harder, really listen, and take proper notice. That is the best way to make sure you are eating right for your own perfectly balanced body/mind/emotional system.

Emotions play a key role in eating, not just because of the pleasure and enjoyment you get when you eat. Food is very comforting. It is designed to be comforting. There is nothing wrong with eating for comfort. It is all part of the wonderful eating-less-but-enjoying-it-more experience. If you come in from the cold, feeling tired and hungry and fed up, would you really prefer to fix yourself a healthy kale salad? Or would you want a warm bowl of soup with crusty bread? Or a dish of hot spicy chili with fluffy rice and a dollop of sour cream on top?

Many years ago, when I was in my early 20s, a great friend of mine taught me an important lesson. I was, of course, always on a diet of some kind. I would eat my permitted food or starve myself, depending on the plan I was following. I was hard on myself. I was strict. I often caved in to temptation. My friend, who was naturally slim, observed my mad habits over many years and listened to my complaints about what foods I was or was not allowed to eat.

She eventually told me this: "You want to eat something, go ahead and eat it. Because after you have eaten your diet food and sipped your herb tea and told yourself how virtuous you are being, your mind will still *want* that food, the one you didn't allow yourself to have. You'll probably eat it anyway. So why don't you go ahead and have that first. Satisfy your desire. Then see what happens."

I think she was eating a bag of lemon sherbet candy at the time, probably her dinner, but never mind that. She was exactly right. Denial doesn't work. In fact, denial can make you feel desperate and, sooner or later, denial will blow your good intentions right out of the water.

HOW TO EAT LESS

"You'll eat foods that you love and give you pleasure, but you'll be satisfied with much less. And your body will thank you for it."
— *Creating a Slim, Healthy Body,* Track 1

Whatever you are eating now you are going to eat less of it but your awareness of the food and the pleasure you're going to enjoy will increase exponentially. Your perception of the amount of food you are eating will change when you approach your meal with a new level of focused attention. It will seem to your mind and body that you are eating the same amount, maybe even more. You'll certainly feel as if you've had a lovely, satisfying eating experience. You'll have enjoyed food that you already like the taste of and that you feel comfortable about eating. But the amount will perhaps be only *half as much*.

I choose this simple and easily quantifiable measure so that you can benchmark what you are doing now against what you did before. It is easy to eat half, and by doing so you'll give yourself a fantastic starting point to fine-tune the amount of food your body really needs. But everyone is an individual, so there is always room for flexibility. Depending on your level of activity, you may need more energy for your lifestyle. The image of a large orange which is an integral part of the verbal guidance, is a useful one to keep in mind. It concentrates the attention and give you a simple concept to work with. The most important part of eating less is the *enjoying it more*.

There is science behind this way of eating. It involves engaging all your senses and making sure that you focus completely on the lovely food. You engage your natural inner systems which govern appetite and hunger and satisfaction.

These systems evolved to help us survive when food had to be hunted or gathered and was the primary focus of everyday life. Appetite is a powerful driver that ensured mankind's survival in times of food scarcity when the available food was dull, bad tasting and may even have been rotten. When eating was a matter of life or death, I don't think our primitive ancestors refused any food, no matter how horrible it tasted. Therefore appetite and hunger, driving us to eat to survive, has its roots in humankind's distant past.

YOUR APPETITE IS REGULATED BY "HARD WIRING"

We might imagine a sort of hard wiring (made up of nerves and chemical switches) that connects the mind, the eyes, the nose, mouth and tongue and the stomach. The bloodstream is involved, monitoring blood glucose and hormone levels. This natural system drives humans to want to eat when survival is at stake. In the distant past, if there was only a bowl of leftover gruel for supper, a lump of stale bread or a bland dish of greasy potage (a kind of medieval vegetable stew), our ancestors would still want to eat it, even if it tasted horrible.

With these ideas in mind, imagine the connections between nerves and chemical switches transmitting signals back and forth between the mind, the eyes, the nose, mouth and tongue and the stomach. This complex system evolved to ensure humankind could survive and eat whatever food was available in just the right amounts to maintain wellbeing.

It was also important that our ancestors understood when they had eaten enough. "Enough" would ensure survival until the next meal, whenever that might be. Enough would also ensure food was shared between other group members and not merely eaten by the strongest. Some of the internal messages are transmitted throughout the body using chemical switches, such as the hormones ghrelin and leptin. Ghrelin has been identified as a hunger hormone, traveling via the bloodstream and acting on the hypothalamus to make you want to eat. Leptin has been found to have the opposite effect, signaling fullness and satisfaction and suppressing appetite.

When you eat less but enjoy it more you engage these systems in a natural way. Conversely, if you fail to respect the inner switches, you will have no way of understanding hunger and fullness. Eating less but enjoying it more *automatically* engages these internal biological systems in your favor.

A perfect eating-less-but-enjoying-it-more experience would be like this: A quiet, peaceful space where you will not be disturbed. No distractions of any sort. No phones, laptops, TV, books, magazines, newspapers, radio, conversation or background noise. Track 2 will initially be your companion while you learn this important skill. Otherwise, you can enjoy a little light background music if the silence disturbs you.

The food you prepare is exactly what you want to eat. Your meal takes into account how hungry you are, how active you are and when you will next eat. If you're going to be using a lot of energy later, or there'll be a few extra hours before your next meal, eat a bigger portion. This is not starvation. Consider your meal. How does it relate to your imagined stomach size? Is it about half your normal portion, about the size of a large orange, for example? Recognize the intention to eat the right amount for you to lose weight but feel energized during those "times in between meals."

Sit comfortably and allow yourself time to look at your food. Hopefully you have presented it nicely. Use your eyes to tell your brain it's time to eat. Your brain wakes up and gets all the other senses and digestive organs ready. Your hormone switches begin to trigger hungry feelings inside you.

Smell your food. Let those aromas awaken your appetite. Pick up your cutlery and take a mouthful. Did you know that your lips have more sensory nerve endings than any other area on the body? More than anywhere else! A rough idea would be about 10,000 nerve endings. It's also estimated you have between 5,000 to 10,000 taste buds on your tongue. All ready for you to have a party with that food you are just about to eat. Another interesting bit of science is that taste buds renew themselves every 14 days. You may think that your taste buds are worn out or not particularly sensitive and you don't taste your food with any great level of enjoyment. However, the science says otherwise. Consider the idea that every time you eat, about 10% of your taste buds are tasting the flavor of your food for the *very first time*. Those freshly grown 500 to 1,000 taste buds will be experiencing a never-before experienced flavor-bomb, for the very first time at every meal. Honor and respect your taste buds by giving them great tasting food to eat. That sounds like another excuse for a party!

When you eat, your mission is to get the maximum pleasure out of your food. That involves textures, temperatures, tastes, sweet, sour, bitter, salt and the elusive umami savory flavor that is so delicious. The aroma of the food will also enhance the enjoyment, so keep all your senses engaged with the process. Mix up the ingredients for each mouthful. Try different combinations. Find out what this food really tastes like when you've chewed it over and over. Release the deep flavors and enjoy the layers of pleasure that are revealed.

Repeat. Stay focused. Sip a little water or whatever you are drinking. Are the flavors as expected? Are you surprised how delicious this meal is? Does any of this food disappoint? Does anything on your plate taste different to you? Maybe, if you are eating something you normally enjoy, you find it doesn't live up to your expectations. As you learn to experience food more fully, your likes and dislikes may change. It will be interesting to find out if you prefer to eat different things when you are tasting food properly.

Pay attention to how this food is making you feel. Is it making you feel good inside? How satisfied are you with the experience? How does your stomach feel? Are you noticing any feelings of fullness yet? Pause and pay attention to how full you feel.

And as you practice eating this way, time will slow down for you. Because you are so aware of this wonderful eating experience, it will seem like time is slowing down and you've been enjoying this meal for a long time. The sensation of time slowing down is a completely natural effect of being very focused with no outside distractions. It's part of an interesting state of altered awareness, a light trance, that you will experience when you eat in this way. You will be more awake and aware than if you were distracted while you eat.

As you continue to enjoy your meal, notice again how full you feel. Be aware of your stomach and how the food is gently pressing against your insides. By now, some of that lovely nourishment will be making its way into your bloodstream, firing you up with energy for the next part of your day. As you eat, as you pause to sip your drink, allow yourself to look forward to whatever you are doing next. How can you make the next part of your day more enjoyable? Is there something you could add to your schedule that will improve your day?

After you finish your meal, check your feelings inside. Full and satisfied. Tell this to yourself. Maybe you've planned something nice for dessert, keeping to the same eating-less-but-enjoying-it-more principles. Go ahead and enjoy it.

When you have practiced this skill many times over several weeks, you'll do it without all the thinking, the stages, the concentrating. It will become second nature. Soon it will become automatic, it will be your new habit. You'll do it without putting effort in. It will become your default way of eating. That's good, because then you can relax and know you'll be eating less and losing weight and feeling great.

THE WONDERFUL TIME IN BETWEEN MEALS
When you eat at mealtimes with nothing in between, it opens up a whole world of possibilities. The time in between meals will be when your life truly begins. There's a saying about this: *eat to live or live to eat*. As you'll be eating to live from now on, it makes perfect sense to make those times in between meals as rewarding as possible.

The verbal guidance in Track 1 advises you to "forget about food." That is a freeing statement. You will enjoy this wonderful time when you can be free from all thoughts of food. As I mentioned previously, food can dominate the mental landscape and take over your life. All your thoughts may revolve around food. Your inner dialogue might be dominated by how good you've been or how bad you've been or what you are going to eat next or what you ate a few hours ago or how you're going to resist that donut somebody left on your desk.

Blissful amnesia about food during the time in between meals is another natural by-product of this process. It feels like you are being set free. You can focus on making your life more enjoyable, more worthwhile, maybe get down to some problem solving you've been putting off. Perhaps there is an issue you need to look right in the eye, but until now you've been avoiding it by eating all the time. This is a time to take those next important steps towards building the life you really want.

WHAT DOES HUNGRY FEEL LIKE?

I've heard a myth about losing weight. It seems you can lose weight by only eating when you are hungry. I don't dispute that logical idea, but in 20 years of working with people who've wanted to lose weight but could not, I've noticed hunger is often an alien concept to them. Hunger is not in their vocabulary. That's not necessarily because they haven't been hungry. It's just that people are individuals and it follows that they experience hunger in different ways.

Hunger isn't always a gnawing pain in the stomach, or the feeling of being lightheaded or empty inside. People experience different hunger sensations, sometimes so subtle they cannot easily recognize them.

Hunger can sometimes trigger negative emotions. Hunger can sometimes make you feel weak or fearful or desperate. Your deep inner survival instinct does not want to feel such emotions. While it might seem odd in our modern world that hunger can make a person feel this way, it is totally understandable when you pause to consider what hunger means in the parts of the world where people struggle to get enough to eat.

In humankind's past history, our ancestors would have experienced hunger that spelled a threat to their very existence. It's possible that deep ancestral memories remain inside us, reminding us of those negative emotions associated with hunger. To the subconscious mind, hunger may trigger the thought that your survival is at stake. When you get hungry, your natural response would be to eat something.

When you eat less but enjoy it more there will be times when you notice you are just a little bit hungry for your next meal, enough so you really look forward to eating. When you are a little bit hungry, food tastes even better. It really does. It's almost as if your whole digestive system is designed so that food tastes even more delicious when you feel hungry.

You can increase your enjoyment of food by feeling a little bit hungry before you eat. This way of thinking might not fit in with your own food habits. You may be the kind of person who cannot wait for dinner and has to eat something to stave off the hunger pangs. Pause for a moment and think about how you feel about being hungry.

Depending on what generation you are from, you might recall parents chastising you for "ruining your appetite" by snacking before a meal. When somebody slaved over a hot stove to make your dinner and somebody had to work hard to buy the food in the first place, it's no surprise that eating between meals was frowned upon in the past. Food took up a big chunk of a family's weekly budget. Leaving something uneaten on the plate was likely to result in an argument. Being sent to bed with no supper was a bitter punishment when hunger was keenly felt. Food was an expensive, important resource not to be wasted. Children from that time learned exactly what hunger felt like. I'm not making a case for reliving those times, but I know for a fact that food tastes much, much better when you are a little bit hungry. I wonder if you are curious to find out what I mean.

The exceptions are diabetics or those with any health concern where hunger or low blood sugar is contra-indicated.

Diabetics must manage blood sugar very carefully. Letting blood glucose levels drop is NOT advocated. If you are managing diabetes and you need to maintain stable blood glucose, think about planning one or more snacks to break up the time in between meals. Snacks must be enjoyable, eaten quietly and with maximum pleasure. That is okay. Adjusting meals, ensuring a good balance of nutrients that includes proteins and fats for sustenance, will help keep blood sugar in balance. Diabetics must be guided by their blood sugar readings. I know diabetics are already likely to be experts in this. Losing weight may help with the management of Type 2 diabetes and will also help with diabetes-related health concerns. Support from a health professional will guide you. Further information about good nutrition can be found by visiting the American Diabetes Association website, see the resources section at the end of this book.

Sometimes having a stomach or digestive problem can make feeling hunger very uncomfortable. Therefore, plan to make sure your eating program, meal times and portion sizes are adjusted to minimize any discomfort. Take the advice of your health professional. Gentle weight loss will follow.

The bottom line is: everything you eat must be enjoyed fully. In that way you ensure your inner appetite systems are activated by what you are eating. If you have to eat something that is not a planned meal then you must sit down, savor the food and enjoy every mouthful. Grabbing a snack and eating it in a few mouthfuls will not cancel out the consequence of the snack so go ahead and get the most pleasure out of it. There is no room for deprivation in this plan. There is no cause for discomfort, physical, mental or emotional. Only pleasure and enjoyment are permitted.

THIS METHOD WORKS ON SO MANY LEVELS

If you have always suffered when you've been on a diet, then everything you've read so far will seem unbelievable. But think for a moment. Why should being miserable, eating nasty food and feeling sorry for yourself result in more weight loss? The plain fact is, the *complete opposite* is true. Weight loss happens when you eat what you enjoy, feel great and integrate this easy method into your everyday life. When you are having fun you keep going. It's effortless and enjoyable. You feel better every day. You notice the pounds dissolving. You eat less but you never feel deprived or fed up or sorry for yourself. Your mind simply cannot find a reason to instruct you to give up.

So you keep going a bit longer. You soon realize that you don't want to go back to those old ways of eating, barely tasting your food but eating double the portion size in comparison with what you eat now. You feel empowered. You feel in control of your life. You simply never think about food unless you are preparing it or eating it. Food is relegated (in the nicest possible way) to its rightful place in your life. You eat to live. That's it. End of story.

If you want to speed up your weight loss, and it feels okay, you can eat a bit less. It all depends on what sized portions you gave yourself when you began the program. If you want to slow down your weight loss you can eat a bit more at mealtimes. But you never go back to your old habits. This is a permanent change.

Integrating this way of eating into your everyday lifestyle can be likened to growing strong mental brakes. If you are in the habit of eating all the time or nibbling between meals, you don't have any mental brakes to help you. You don't know how or when to stop eating. Your mind has a permanent "green light means go" sign inside it. With this method you will grow strong brakes. Iron willpower, to put it another way. You can choose to apply those brakes more often or ease up on the brakes from time to time. The important thing is that you now have brakes where none existed before. Surprise yourself with how much you enjoy putting those brakes on.

WHAT IF THE SCALES SHOW I'M NOT LOSING WEIGHT?
How quickly you will lose weight to reveal your slim, healthy body depends on you as a unique individual. You can set the pace. How

quickly you lose your weight is further related to what you are doing now. If you have already lost weight and are on the final pounds, it's normal for things to be slower than if you are at the start of the process with a lot of weight to lose.

All this you probably know already. The most important thing is to get the eating-less-but-enjoying-it-more skill embedded deeply in your subconscious mind so it becomes your habit, your default way of eating. Once this is in place, you can fine-tune the process. You can tweak the amount of food you eat or decide to focus more on adjusting the types of foods you eat. This evolution might happen on its own. Your body may send you messages about eating more healthy foods. While I shun the idea of foods being good or bad, you may find reworking your balance of different foods and food groups pays off. You must enjoy yourself, however. There must be no skimping on pleasure.

The *Metabolism Boost* and *Iron Willpower* tracks will serve you well while you make adjustments to the foods you eat and enjoy. You will then discover that the scales respond to these adjustments and show you the results you wish for.

A word about the scales. They are your friend. They tell you what you need to know so you can make those fine adjustments, if necessary. The idea that you should throw the scales away doesn't fit with your new confidence and self control. You can look at what the scales say and use that information intelligently to inform your choices.

Make sure the scales are good ones, accurate and user-friendly. You need to have confidence in what the scales are telling you. I once worked with a partially-sighted gentleman who needed to lose a lot of weight to help him improve his health and mobility. We decided to find him some talking scales. He made me laugh when he said that the scales often told him: "One person at a time, please."

THE REVELATION OF CHANGING TASTES

When you really taste what you eat it's hard to enjoy flavors that are not 100% delicious. It's difficult to enjoy food that tastes of things that nature hasn't produced, such as the exotic chemicals included in the ingredients list of factory produced food. Remember how sensitive your taste buds are, how alive with nerve endings your lips are. You may find you don't quite enjoy the same food as you used to.

As you listen to your body and give it what it likes and needs, you may discover you prefer food that isn't dusted with chemicals. It hurts me to say that, as I honestly believe you and I must eat exactly *what we love*. But there are some eating experiences that can only be endured when you bolt the food down without tasting it. For that reason, you are urged to be open-minded about what your newly-awakened taste buds tell you is delicious and what your taste buds tell you is nasty.

An example: an avocado, lightly seasoned with salt and black pepper. That's all I'm going to say. Taste it and find out what I'm talking about. Or try strawberries with a sprinkle of vanilla sugar, then taste the strawberries with a splash of balsamic vinegar. Compare the eating enjoyment between a cheap bar of chocolate and a few squares of a high quality brand.

There are no recipes in this book or advice about food groups or what is good or bad or what fits in with government guidelines. I believe our bodies will tell us exactly what is good for us to eat and to lose weight. You will easily be able to work with any personal food preferences or any intolerances or allergies. Commit now to listening to what your body tells you about what it wants you to eat.

It is recommended that you enjoy the experiments with different foods that follow at the end of this chapter. Make it into a game. Compare six different kinds of chocolate or cheese or whatever you love. Really discover which of the many different types of food taste best to you.

TWO CAUTIONARY TALES

A woman once told me her story about something that happened when she experienced eating less but enjoying it more. The story has stuck with me, as it did with her.

She was at work, practicing her eating-less-but-enjoying-it-more routine quietly and peacefully at her desk. She had prepared a packed lunch. She assured me it was delicious. A few desks away sat two colleagues who were also eating at their desks. They were talking to each other and looking at their computer screens. She observed them stuffing huge chunks of food into their mouths and swallowing the food without tasting. Their jaws were working overtime and they were talking as they chewed.

This lady couldn't help noticing how indifferent her workmates were to their lunches. She realized, as she looked at them, that she would never go back to her old ways of eating without thinking. Without warning, her mind then morphed the two colleagues into two hogs at a trough, gorging themselves. Not that there is anything wrong with hogs because they are beautiful creatures. But not necessarily in an office environment.

Her mind had shown her a powerful picture that was a symbol of what she was leaving behind. That image stayed with her and she mentioned it often. Suffice it to say, she lost all her excess weight and regained her happy life.

A few years ago there was rash of diet shows on TV involving overweight people who were competing to lose the most pounds, while undertaking various challenges, gym routines and punishing physical activities. The winner of one particular series was a man who had lost the most weight. He was interviewed on camera, discussing what changes he had made to his diet. During his talk, he held in his hand a tray of sushi. As he spoke about how much he had changed, he threw the sushi rolls into his mouth like peanuts and swallowed each one down in a single gulp. He continued talking to the interviewer as he did so, chomping on the food and swallowing it without tasting. He explained to the camera how he used to eat candy like that, a whole box a time, but now he had substituted sushi. He believed this habit change had caused him to lose the most weight and win the show.

I felt very sad. The contestants in the show had endured all those weeks of struggle and not one of the many doctors or psychologists or personal trainers had thought to teach the contestants how to eat and enjoy their food properly. Everyone involved had focused on the type of food that was eaten, labeling foods good and bad, pushing the notion that the only way to lose weight was to give up delicious foods and undertake hours of strenuous exercise.

That TV interview is another memory that stays with me. It reinforces what I understand about how to balance eating delicious food, having maximum pleasure and enjoyment, with creating a slim, healthy body for life. That is how I know this method is just right, neither extreme, nor punishing, nor unpleasant, nor unsustainable. This program takes the healthy middle way. Designed to fit everyone, but respecting that each person is a unique individual.

FREQUENTLY ASKED QUESTIONS

WHY DO YOU SAY THIS IS AN ENJOYABLE CHALLENGE?

Think about how eating behavior has changed during the last 50 years. It used to be socially unacceptable to eat in the street, or anywhere other than at a dining table. Now you can eat anywhere without people staring at you. Literally anytime and anywhere. But do you ever notice people (at home or work or in restaurants or in the street) who are concentrating *completely* on their food? I doubt it. Twenty years ago, people ate TV dinners. Their minds were absorbed in whatever was on the TV, while their bodies ate food without tasting it or enjoying it. Today, look in any restaurant and notice tables of diners, all glued to their smart phones while spooning food into their mouths without noticing anything about it.

How difficult will it be if you need to break these habits? I estimate it will be a real challenge but, once you've got the hang of it and enjoyed the wonderful rewards, you'll never want to distract yourself again.

If you didn't have this guided meditation to teach and support you, you might never be able to learn how to do it. Yet, as you immerse yourself in this experience (and have lots of fun with your food along the way), soon you won't need to have complete peace and quiet to help you focus on your food. You will give food your full attention automatically. There will be happy restaurant outings, great family dinners, gossipy lunches with friends, all the while eating less but enjoying it more. You will have learned to focus all your attention on the food while you are eating it. Your mind and body will be in tune with this process. You'll have full awareness of the lovely food, and your body will signal when it's time to stop eating. Of course, while you are practicing this new eating challenge (and ignoring your phone or whatever is your particular distraction), there will be plenty of enjoyment to be had from the food.

WHAT IF I CAN'T MANAGE ON SMALLER PORTIONS?

This way of eating grows stronger with every day, and every time you listen to the guided meditation track. It is cumulative. It is also flexible. You can therefore decrease your portion sizes slowly. You can go at a comfortable pace. The only rules I'd recommend not to be broken are:

- You may not eat anything you do not like. Leave it on your plate or throw it away.
- You must focus all your attention on eating.

- You should not eat between meals, allowing you to grow those important mental "brakes."
- If you do *need* to snack between meals you must sit down, eat slowly and enjoy every bite. That's an order!

With these simple rules in place, I'm confident you'll be eating less food in no time. How much less will depend on how you feel and how fast you want to lose weight. Fast isn't necessarily good, however.

WHAT IS THE MOST IMPORTANT PART OF THIS PROGRAM?

There are lot of different tracks and you may wonder what to prioritize. The most important element that will make you lose weight is eating less but enjoying it more. Therefore, Tracks 1 and 2 should be your primary focus for about 28 days. It's been estimated that it takes this length of time to break an old habit and make a new one. You will know when this method becomes your default way of eating. Once this habit is successfully "installed" it will carry you through all of life's ups and downs and ensure you keep enjoying your food and losing weight. If this part of the program is not thoroughly embedded in your subconscious mind, if you skip doing your practice and start doing other things like the absorbing track *Metabolism Boost*, for example, you'll not enjoy the benefits of having this method as your automatic default way of eating. You'll have to keep trying at every mealtime. I want this way of eating and losing weight to be effortless and to become your natural routine. I reaffirm the necessity to get this eating-less-but-enjoying-it-more habit totally set in your subconscious mind like a block of concrete. Then you can add in other tracks and enjoy the journey of self discovery as you progress.

Make up your mind to give this program 100%; make it your number one priority and you'll get to enjoy all that lovely food while you do so. You might imagine yourself to be a top restaurant critic, destined to eat gourmet food in all the best places, and then writing a glowing (or damning) review about your dining experience. Have high standards. Settle only for the finest cuisine. Give your meal marks out of 10 for deliciousness. Keep a notebook. You can then look back at your journey and notice how you developed, how your tastes changed, how your attitudes to eating changed, how you learned to love eating and weren't afraid to say so out loud.

HOW IS IT POSSIBLE TO SLOW DOWN TIME?

Time distortion is when time seems to speed up or slow down depending on your perception of it. This tells us that time has a *subjective* element. Have you noticed how long 30 minutes at the dentist's seems? Or how quickly a thrilling sports event progresses? When you are bored, the clock ticks by with agonizing slowness. When you are already late for an appointment, time whizzes by too fast.

Time is a strange phenomenon. Have you ever wondered if it is actually real? Perhaps that sounds a bit esoteric. However, consider the philosophical idea that there is really only *now*. Now is real time when you inhabit the fullness of your being with no regression into past memories or progression into possible future events. Now can then expand and take over. You can be totally present and take part in your life as it's happening in this very moment.

As the average human mind lives mostly in the past or the future, flitting restlessly between these mental states, the potential joy of being fully in the present is lost. Learning mastery of time will yield unexpected benefits. What if you could slow down that moment of perfect enjoyment so it lasted for much longer in your perception? And conversely, what if those times at the dentist's could speed up? Time is elastic, so they say. With practice you can make time very elastic.

HOW CAN I FORGET ABOUT FOOD?

If food is on your mind all the time you may wonder how you can change this. Given the right support, however, your mind will easily accept the suggestion to forget about food between meals. It's almost as if your mind is waiting to receive the instruction. The messages within the tracks will facilitate this sense of forgetting. When you begin to enrich your time in between meals with wonderful, exciting, fulfilling activities, food will be the last thing you want to think about until it's time to eat again.

WHAT ADVICE CAN YOU GIVE ABOUT EATING OUT?

Eating out is a great way to test your mastery of this eating-less-but-enjoying-it-more skill. As you sit down at your table, notice how in control you feel. The menu describes the delicious foods you will enjoy. You now have a real challenge, to decide which is the most enjoyable dish; what menu choice is really going to give you the most pleasure. You may decide to focus your attention on enjoying only one course. Or you may wish to try two or three courses. You may decide to share a plate of food with your companion. Restaurants sometimes have menu items you can order as either a starter or a main course, giving you the choice of enjoying two smaller dishes while allowing you to eat only the right amount of food to make you feel satisfied.

With your new, more streamlined stomach size, do not overestimate how much food you can eat. The phrase: "having eyes bigger than your belly," comes to mind. It can be frustrating to be part way through a starter and sense the "full up" signal from your stomach. Of course, you can choose to leave some food on your plate to allow full enjoyment of your next course. Take-out bags are also useful if this happens to you. Let eating out be a good learning experience for you.

Eating out can feel like an emotional minefield for many overweight people. Some people might feel judged and this is a reaction many overweight diners have told me about. They feel judged by other diners or by their own critical inner selves. They feel compelled to choose a small salad to signal to the restaurant that they *know* they need to lose weight. If they choose a dish that they want to eat, it's impossible to be seen to enjoy it. You can now decide to let go of those feelings, secure in the knowledge you are on track and you are in control. Ignore the inner critic because that person no longer has any power over you. Also ignore everyone else who may or may not be looking at you.

Buffets and family gatherings can present a different kind of challenge. The food is there and it stays there, in plain sight. A recall a woman told me such events were her worst nightmare. "I'm not safe around a buffet," she said. Years of experience have taught me something about buffet food. It all looks very tempting when you look at it, spread out abundantly along the table. But some dishes taste much better than others. Appearances can be very deceptive.

You have your new streamlined stomach size, therefore it's vital you choose the most delicious food to eat. Either take a tiny taster-sized portion of several dishes and check for deliciousness before making your decision, or be prepared to try something and decide it's not as wonderful to eat as it looks. You will have to leave it and get something else. Be fussy. Always wait a while before any second trip to the buffet. Notice the fullness in your stomach first. You will not want to feel stuffed and uncomfortable later, when the dancing begins.

I FEEL LIKE A DIETING FAILURE, HOW CAN I OVERCOME THIS?
Does your past experience of trying to lose weight make you feel like a failure? It's perfectly possible to start a weight loss diet every day, then give up by dinner time. Over and over again. That's a lot of giving up. However many times you have tried unsuccessfully to lose weight, or partially succeeded and not followed through, please understand *this does not matter one bit*. It is irrelevant. You simply did not have the resources you required to reach your goal. This program contains a complete package of everything you need. Failure wears away at your sense of self and your confidence. Your mind sends you negative messages that pervade your thoughts imprinting the belief that you are a

dieting failure and you'll never succeed. That's when your mind tells you to stop trying. Not trying is another way of saying, "I'm scared I'll fail again and I couldn't stand that, so I'll make my excuses and not make any effort. If I do fail, I can console myself I didn't really try. My fragile self confidence will remain intact."

Are you a person who doesn't give their all, in case you fail? You'd be surprised how normal this behavior is. It's an example of the protective influence of your subconscious mind. This idea is explored further in later chapters to help you understand how your mind works both for you but sometimes against you. Your subconscious mind is determined to prevent you getting to rock bottom in case you never get out of it. *Not trying* is a clever way that protects you from facing the potentially devastating consequences of knowing you have failed when you gave it your all. If you only gave 50%, you can console yourself that you can try again another time and you might succeed. Your sense of self is not damaged.

However, if you are in the habit of not giving 100% to anything you do, you will seriously undermine all your efforts to create a slim, healthy body. Everything has been carefully designed to support you on your journey. This program contains 100% effort. It is not half-hearted. It is complete, thorough, tough, gentle, supporting, nourishing, powerful, energizing, confidence-building, healing, and ultimately filled to bursting with the potential for success. Why oh why wouldn't you want to give this program your all, your 100%? Why wouldn't you try?

If you recognize this description and suspect you won't try in case you fail, you must commit to using Track 8, *Release the Past* and Track 9, *Self-Sabotage* to undo all of your learned behaviors. Everything in this program is perfect for you to succeed this time. But you will have to try. There will be no progress for you if these tracks remain in their wrappers. There are no brownie points for having them gathering dust on the shelf, or in a playlist somewhere on your music player, unused.

EATING LESS BUT ENJOYING IT MORE IN PRACTICE

Now you can be the scientist! What are your favorite foods? What, in your view, has the most flavor and gives the most pleasure out of all the different foods that you love to eat?

The following exercise is designed to enhance your experience and show you how sensitive your natural food tasting equipment is. You will engage all your senses which give you the ability to smell, taste, feel and explore all the deliciousness in the food.

Take six cubes or spoonfuls of different foods that you already enjoy and ensure you choose a variety of different flavors and textures so you get the most out of this experiment. An example:

Cheese	Apple	Peanut butter	Chocolate	Natural full-fat yogurt	Fruit preserve

Approach each food and use your eyes to explore the appearance of the food. Then smell the food and wake up your taste buds. When you are ready, taste the food, savoring it fully. Keep tasting until there is no flavor left in your mouth. Have a drink of water, then try the next item.

Make notes as you go along. Find out how many words you can use to describe each food. Rate each food between one to 10. Understand you are exercising your eating equipment to keep it in good shape.

Try other combinations of flavors and textures. You can experiment with different tastes that you don't normally eat:

Bread and butter	A ripe tomato	Honey	A potato chip	Ice cream	A crisp lettuce leaf

Another time you might choose some foods that have some of those exotic chemicals in them — processed factory-produced food. This is so you can compare your experiences and test for deliciousness. Find out exactly how the individual foods taste when you really let all the flavors develop in your mouth. Be open-minded and discerning about how the processing of the food affects your enjoyment.

I once went to try out for a food tasting program. It was a voluntary position as part of a panel. I live close to a huge multi-national food company that makes many popular brands of food. The company was recruiting food tasters to try out new products at the development stage. We were all tested to find out how sensitive our palates were. The test food item? Water. All different varieties of water from many sources. It was fascinating to use my taste buds so effectively that I could differentiate the flavor nuances within the many different varieties of water that I was offered. I learned exactly how sensitive my taste buds were. You can also try this experiment at home with different types of water.

Follow this food tasting exercise with the next chapter which is about practicing eating less but enjoying it more while you are in the waking state. You eat your meal while listening to Track 2, the guided meditation for use with your eyes open, fully awake and aware of your eating experience. Using Track 2 in conjunction with Track 1 will speed up your progress and ensure you are fully immersed in the core elements of this program.

CHAPTER 2
EATING LESS BUT ENJOYING IT MORE
WAKING MEDITATION

Eating less but enjoying your food more is an amazing skill to learn. When you practice, you'll be awakening the deep part of yourself that knows how to create a loving, harmonious and respectful relationship with food.

This track is designed to be a practical meditation that you do with your eyes open and all your consciousness in the "now." You will still journey into an altered state of relaxation, but you will focus fully on your food, allow distractions to fade, and gain maximum pleasure from your eating experience. You will also take great care in the choosing, preparation, and presentation of your meal.

This track is accompanied by Hemi-Sync® tones comprising an opening melody followed by pink noise which is designed to lead you into the best state of awareness to achieve the maximum benefits.

It is perfectly possible to eat delicious food every day of your life and never experience 100% awareness of doing so. Typical distractions include fiddling with your phone, flipping through a magazine, watching TV, talking to your companions, working, doing your emails, or doing whatever you think is more important than focusing 100% on the meal in front of you.

WORKING WITH YOUR NATURAL APPETITE REGULATORS

These distractions create an interesting dilemma for your mind. It wants and needs to know you have eaten enough to sustain you throughout your day, yet it isn't aware you have eaten enough because it has been so busy messaging your friends. Therefore it keeps the "hungry switch" firmly in the "on" position, and you carry on eating because you have no idea whether you are full or not. You may get to the end of your meal, look down at your empty plate or crumpled sandwich wrapper and feel thoroughly cheated. You may feel as if you hardly tasted anything. And inside, you still feel hungry.

This is a guaranteed recipe for overeating. And it could be happening at every meal, every day of your life.

Do you often get this feeling that you are not satisfied with your meals? Is it normal for you to go back for a second helping, or move on to grazing on desserts or snacks? The evidence is there, all over your body. You *are* getting enough to eat, yet your mind and your stomach beg to differ with that opinion. In their view, you hardly eat a thing. At least, not that you are aware of. Take a moment to remember yest-erday's meals. What you ate and how you ate it. Estimate how much of your attention you devoted to your food.

I know what it's like to be in a rush and grab something easy and portable to eat in the car on my way to appointment (that I'm probably late for). I have encountered people who eat a bowl of cereal standing at the kitchen counter, shoveling the food down so they can minimize the time it takes to eat it. A walk down any street in any city will yield numerous examples of people chomping on takeout food as they walk along. All this fast food is bypassing the natural appetite regulators of the human system. This is the hard-wired automatic system that registers when you are eating. This regulation system unlocks the chemical switches that turn appetite on and off again when you have eaten enough, thereby giving you a feeling of fullness and satisfaction. In order to eat less and reveal the slim you inside, you must fully engage this system and use it to your advantage. Otherwise you'll end up feeling hungry, unsatisfied, deprived, and unhappy (again). You know what happens when a new eating plan makes you feel that way. You give up.

The main core track of this program, Track 1, is your blueprint for changing your eating habits and turning yourself into an unstoppable slimming phenomenon. This waking meditation allows you to practice this skill "live" and become expert at it. Once you have this skill installed and working at full efficiency, you will never again be able to overeat because you aren't focusing 100% on your food. Your natural, automatic appetite regulators will work to optimize the amount of food you eat for fullness and satisfaction, and you will lose weight as a result. You will never feel deprived.

HOW TO USE THIS WAKING MEDITATION
Begin by preparing something you really want to eat. Make sure you are hungry. Food always tastes more delicious when pangs of hunger make your senses come alive.

Begin this exercise at a time when you are not rushing to get on with the next part of your day. Choose a place to eat where you won't be disturbed, and where other people won't seek you out to distract you. When you are learning this skill, you'll want to be alone when you eat. It may only be for a week or so, then you can rejoin normal meal times. However, it makes sense to give this learning stage your best effort. You are putting your needs first. Be firm with your companions or loved ones. Your health and welfare are at stake. Don't let yourself be persuaded by the argument that it's unsociable to eat alone.

Make this a special occasion. Sit at the table, if you can. Would this experience be more enjoyable with a tablecloth, placemat and your best dishes and cutlery? When you have the food in front of you, plug in your headphones and begin listening to the instructions. This is a ritual of pleasure. Every time you work at this you will make wonderful discoveries about the enjoyment of eating.

You begin by taking a minute to notice everything about your food and honor the earth's bounty in providing it for you.

"Now focus all your attention on the food and notice everything about it, the colors and textures, the appealing presentation. Then lean in and smell the aromas, really wake up all your senses. Signal to your whole body to be ready to eat."
— *Eating Less but Enjoying it More Waking Meditation,* Track 2

The background music and Hemi-Sync® tones that you experience during the eating process have been specifically designed to support your state of focused awareness. Allow yourself to be absorbed into the experience. Imagine you are a top restaurant critic, tasting the food of a celebrity Michelin-starred chef. Perhaps what you are eating is a more humble meal than you would find on a restaurant menu, yet when you uncover layer after layer of flavor and enjoyment, it will seem as though you are enjoying a meal in a fine restaurant. You experience the aromas and flavors of your food through your sense of smell and your sense of taste. Your sense of smell detects the aromatics, the particles of scented air that your food is releasing. Your tongue detects the combinations of sweet and salt, sour and bitter, and the elusive fifth flavor profile which is called umami.

Chefs are always talking about umami. Based on the Japanese idea of savoriness, it can be found in roasted meats, cheese, mushrooms, miso and savory broths, fermented sauces (such as fish sauce) and also potatoes and carrots. If you prefer savory foods, you may have this preference from birth. Researchers have identified the amino acid glutamate, which is responsible for the umami taste, in human breast milk.

As you eat, your mind is focused on what you're doing. With every mouthful, your mind is learning this new skill of 100% focus on your food. Every time you practice, you signal to your mind that you want it to design and install a new subconscious program to adopt this way of eating permanently and make it automatic. Your mind already designs and installs these subconscious programs all the time, whenever you are learning a new skill. Because you are an intelligent being with a massive supercomputer inside your head, you have the capability to write your own software. This new way of eating must supersede your old habit of gobbling food without paying attention to it. Therefore, the learning must be sufficiently compelling to instruct your mind to uninstall the old subconscious program and install this shiny new one instead. That is why you are practicing. Plus it's fun to eat this way; much more fun than many things you can do in life.

You'll be designing and growing a new subconscious program to replace the old one — your old habit of *eating food without thinking*, without focusing all your awareness on your meal. All it takes to design and absorb this software into your mind is for you to listen to the meditations regularly and then practice, practice, practice (which will be relaxing and enjoyable). Your subconscious mind will then do the hard work for you. At the end of this chapter there are some practical examples of how your mind designs and installs its own subconscious programs, so you can benchmark your own experiences and under-stand how powerful that supercomputer in your head really is.

I hope you can now understand why it's so vital to give this method your best endeavor. If you waver and go back to your old ways every now and again, your mind will raise an error message. It will think: "What exactly does my person want me to do? Am I still working on this new subconscious program? Or should I get the old one out of the recycle bin and use that instead?" Understand that you need to keep the instructions to your mind clear and unequivocal. If you tolerate any mixed messages, your mind will not write you a perfect program that you can use to make this way of eating *easy and automatic*.

As you progress with your meal, the verbal guidance prompts you to focus on how full you are becoming. After giving 100% awareness to your eating experience, you now bring your stomach into your bubble of focus. It may take a little more concentration to sense your stomach fully, but as you eat you will increase your ability to feel how the food is making you feel inside.

"Have a sense of how your stomach feels. Be aware of how full and satisfied it feels right now. Your stomach is about the size of a large orange, give or take. That is the optimum size of your meal so that you can be satisfied and properly nourished and have plenty of energy while you lose weight."
— *Eating Less but Enjoying it More Waking Meditation,* Track 2

Work on sensing your feelings of fullness. Be confident you have all the right equipment inside to do this. Sometimes it takes a bit of practice to gather all your awareness and then beam it into your digestive system. You can prompt your mind by placing your hand on your solar plexus area and pressing. Become aware of how the food you've eaten is gently pressing on the insides of your stomach. Estimate how satisfied you feel. In our family we call it "the full-up sign." It comes on when you're close to the point where you can't eat any more.

The image of a large orange is useful to help visualize the optimum size of your stomach. I do mean a large orange, one of those whoppers you get from a really fine harvest. If you are a large person with a demanding physical job who needs more calories than the average, make your orange as large as you need to. But it's still an orange.

Minds like having simple images to act as visual reminders. It will store the idea of this perfect meal size as a neat, colorful picture. If you dislike oranges or they don't agree with your digestion, or if your mind rebels at the thought of having an orange inside you, choose another symbol. Select a symbol that your mind can feel comfortable about.

As you practice eating less and enjoying it more, your stomach will adjust to a natural healthy size. You will then choose to eat this amount of food to satisfy this new stomach size. I have included the statement: "And it may be only *half* of what you have eaten in the past" to give you a clear indication of what to aim for. "Half" is an easy amount of food to visualize and to measure. You can work with this idea and experiment with how it makes you feel. Does eating half leave you satisfied? Do you feel the sweet spot of fullness when you eat only half of what you ate before? Feeling full does not mean feeling like you are going to burst and that you need to undo the button on your waistband. It is a subtle, sweet sensation, associated with comfort, contentment and a sense of energy.

In contrast, when you have eaten so much you are stuffed to bursting, you are likely to feel fatigued, uncomfortable and bloated. It's preferable to prepare a reasonably-sized meal and eat all of it while enjoying it fully, than to make a large meal and leave half on your plate. Many people feel averse to wasting food, and this can compel them to eat more than they want or need.

As you practice eating in this quiet, meditative way, your sense of focus will be completely on your food and your enjoyment of it. You will lose a sense of time. Time will seem to slow down for you because you are only aware of the "now" that is your focused state of attention. This is a good thing. Your mind enjoys the sense of timelessness. As a result it will seem like you have been eating for much longer than the clock tells you. Time distortion is a natural, pleasurable effect of all meditative states, so go ahead and make the most of it.

When you have finished your meal, pause to think about the rest of your day, that special "time in between meals" when you can forget about food. Experiencing the freedom from all thoughts of food will open up exciting new possibilities for you. You can use the same state of focused attention you are learning to enrich many other aspects of your life. You don't have to make dramatic changes. Your life will gently evolve and improve when you give everything you do more focus and consideration.

"The time in between meals now expands and fills up with activities that make you feel alive. Between meals is going to become your special time for yourself, a time when you can really enjoy yourself, really find out what you love doing, what makes your life special and worthwhile."

— *Eating Less but Enjoying it More Waking Meditation*, Track 2

During the times between meals, you'll have more energy to devote to making your life better. It's likely you'll also have a better relationship with time. If you are someone who rushes around, squeezing as much activity as possible into your day, you may find that you approach your schedule with more clarity, with calmer breathing, and with less associated stress. You may think about prioritizing some activities and dropping others. A good exercise is to write down exactly what your priorities are. What aspects of your life would you love to have more time for? How much time, exactly? Thinking about food all the time and fretting about your weight is very time consuming. It makes sense that there will now be more time for you to make your life how you want it to be.

Challenge yourself to write down 10 ways you would like your life to improve. Then write down the ways you can influence those improvements. Divide your improvement plan into small, manageable chunks. Give yourself three of these chunks to work on for a week at a time. Enjoy finding out how easy it is to change.

Your loved ones, family, friends, and colleagues will all benefit from your full attention and the extra time you will devote to them. Even though you will be eating quietly and peacefully without disturbance for a few weeks in the beginning, you will soon graduate to enjoying sociable meals out, family dinners, coffee breaks with colleagues, and all manner of food-related activities that will give you an opportunity to eat less, enjoy it more and have fun with the people you care about.

 If you are obliged to eat with people you don't care about or who would normally stress you out, this is your chance to breathe deep and center yourself, be in the moment and call in your wise inner self to be your companion. The discomfort you might normally experience from such mealtime events will dissolve when you focus your awareness inside. And your wise inner self is always very good company.

You end this track having spent your mealtime in resourceful meditation with your food. You'll feel relaxed but energized. This quiet time to yourself may be a welcome break during a busy day, or you can think of it as a special treat that you give yourself. Every time you practice, you lay down another strong layer of self-belief. You strengthen the subconscious program inside your mind. You make eating less but enjoying it more your personal truth. Your journey towards a slim, healthy body is progressing beautifully.

As you finish eating and turn the track off, your mind will now be focused on what comes next. With an inner feeling of satisfaction and your body nourished properly, you can now forget about food until it's time for your next meal.

YOUR MIND AS A SOFTWARE DESIGNER
I have referred several times to your subconscious mind and the programs that run inside it. It's interesting to think about how this applies to you. It helps to have insight into how your behaviors have developed, how the way you act as a unique person is influenced by

the software inside your mind, much of which you have written yourself, even if you didn't know you were doing it.

Consider the act of learning to walk. This is something that children learn when they are about 12-18 months old. Walking is a very complex activity, involving many nerve signals, muscles, a sense of balance, and multiple sequences of movements. Yet children learn how to do this by observing other people in their environment, and developing the necessary program to carry out this complex series of movements. Children can accomplish this with such a degree of accuracy that they can soon balance on their little squidgy feet, then propel themselves at speed across a room. Observing a child walking for the first time is a joy to behold.

When children are almost ready to walk, they will have observed how it is done and their minds are already designing the software. There may even be a basic template they use, already located in the brain, ready to be activated. Then they begin to practice. They pull themselves up to their feet and experiment with balancing. They hold on to furniture or parents' hands and try over and over to find the balance point while moving from foot to foot.

A child's mind is processing all this data and using it to fine-tune the program being written to make it more effective. All of this is happening inside the subconscious mind, out of ordinary awareness. You cannot try to make new software grow; it happens automatically in response to whatever your learning or development needs are.

I challenge you now to think about a new skill you have learned recently. A popular example is learning to drive. Alternatively, you may have learned how to play a sport, a musical instrument, to speed-read, knit, or put together flat-packed furniture. All these examples share the beginning point: that you *do not* have the ability to do the task.

In the example of learning to drive, you begin by using your logical conscious mind to do all the work. This is the part of your mind that can follow instructions, make decisions, and use judgment. It is awake when you are awake, and is the partner of your subconscious mind.

However, when you are learning to drive you don't have a subconscious program to carry out all the complex sequences of movements and actions required to drive a car. Therefore, your conscious mind has to try and process everything you need to do. It is estimated that your conscious mind, while very powerful at reasoning, only has the processing capacity for working on five to nine thoughts at the same time. As more thoughts have to be processed, other thoughts drop out of focus. And this is what can happen:

You are sitting in the car for the first or second time. Whoever is teaching you instructs you to follow a certain sequence. (This is for a manual transmission).

- Adjust your seat.
- Check that your mirrors are positioned correctly.
- Check that the car is in neutral gear.
- Hands on the steering wheel.
- Turn the key in the ignition or press the start button.
- Now depress the clutch.
- Put the car into gear.
- Check mirrors front and back.
- Signal you are going to move off.
- Release the handbrake.
- Slowly raise the clutch until you feel it bite.
- Simultaneously depress the accelerator (or gas pedal).
- Check the mirrors again.
- Move off and steer the car into the road.

If you count up these actions you'll find there are 14 thoughts to get to that point of moving the car out into traffic. If you can recall your own experience when learning to drive, it's likely you came unstuck at the part where you have to raise the clutch while pressing the gas pedal. That's when you stalled the car. I know I did, many times. I was so bad at it that one time I drained the battery. Every time I stalled I had to turn the engine off and start the whole process again. I thought I'd never get it right. It seemed impossible to do all the actions at the same time.

After you have successfully driven out into the traffic, it gets even more complicated. Once you've gotten onto the road, you have to work out how to change gears, slow down, speed up, signal, negotiate traffic lights, junctions, roundabouts and follow directions to get you to your destination.

But all this time — when your stress levels are through the roof and your mind is struggling to drive the car safely on the highway — your subconscious mind is very busy. It's processing all the data about driving and designing a program for you to carry out all the small repetitive processes that are part of driving automatically. Within a few weeks of practice you can move off without stalling the car. You change gear without thinking. You slow down when you see brake lights come on in front of you. You are able to judge distances when you're in moving traffic and make turns without crashing into an oncoming car. This happens because your subconscious mind has designed and installed a subconscious program for you to use. This leaves your conscious mind with the free space to notice road signs, be aware of other vehicles, spot upcoming hazards, and drive safely.

Do you now have an insight into how amazing and powerful your mind is? If you are someone who loves the latest electronic gadget or gets excited about new technology, take a moment to respect the computing power that lives inside your head. It's estimated we only use 10-20% of our brain's capabilities. I'm awestruck when I think about the potential we might unleash to do great things if we could learn how to harness our innate mental power and turn it to good. Throughout this program there are references to your conscious mind and your subconscious mind. These terms help us to comprehend the myriad complexities of the "supercomputer" inside your head.

Conscious mind — Awake and aware, has judgment, decision making capability, opinions, and logical thought. It has a sense of what is right and wrong, good and bad. It likes to categorize things and make sense of them.

Subconscious mind — On duty 24 hours a day, the data repository, the location of your memories, software programs, and belief systems. The imagination exists in this part of the mind. Dreams are created here. The subconscious is benign in that it does not judge the data. It has no sense of right and wrong, good and bad. It organizes the data so the conscious mind can make sense of it.

This model also links to the information about brain wave frequencies in the chapter about Hemi-Sync® at the end of this book. You can explore how your brain waves resonate through Beta, Alpha, Theta and Delta wavelengths and the brain states associated with them.

The aim of this simple model is to help you to make sense of the life changes you want to make to achieve your slim, healthy body for life. Whatever is happening now inside your mind, it is going to change. The influences for these changes will come from the 12 tracks in this album. Your subconscious mind will then design and install the necessary software, using the suggestions in the album as new data for you to work with. Your conscious mind will utilize the programs to manifest your slim, healthy body and make it into your reality.

When I think about the mind, I don't imagine it living inside my brain. I consider the brain to be the hardware, the equipment. I think of my mind and its thoughts existing in an energy cloud around my head However, you can interpret this idea in any way that is right for you.

CHAPTER 3
IRON WILLPOWER

"Deep inside you there is a well of strength that you can call on to make those life changes that you desire — a slim, healthy body filled with the pure joy of being alive — and to do this you are going to develop iron willpower."

— *Iron Willpower,* Track 3

When you begin a plan to lose weight, your energy is high, you are full of ideas and positive motivation and losing weight is your top priority. However, over time these feelings fade. The eating plan is no longer new and interesting. The scales refuse to budge. You are surrounded by temptation. A voice inside your head keeps telling you to give up. Your life is full of stress and pressure, and you don't have the time you need to devote to your diet plan. Besides, there is a huge slice of chocolate fudge cake in the fridge and it's got your name on it.

What you need is a strong dose of iron willpower, sufficient to carry you forward with unbreakable resolve. This Hemi-Sync® track will do just that. It will build up a burning core of fiery willpower inside you. You'll never weaken again. Iron willpower will carry you effortlessly through all the ordinary ups and downs of life and ensure you feel as fresh, strong and motivated on day 79 as you did on day 1.

WILLPOWER VERSUS WON'T POWER

Before we discuss what willpower is and how it works, let's consider for a moment the thoughts and feelings associated with wanting to giving up your diet and go back to your old ways of eating. It's always wise to get up close and personal with your "enemy." We need to square up to these thoughts and feelings and understand them better. I nicknamed these thoughts and feelings "won't power" which is a neat way of describing the opposite of willpower.

Have you noticed that your mind has a habit of twittering on in the background, providing a sort of negative commentary about whatever you are doing? It may be that you've become so used to having this mental background music you have stopped listening carefully to what it says. It's a bit like the music played in shopping malls, you soon learn to ignore it. Your mind chatters on about won't power using language that is designed to undermine you.

I wonder what the words your mind uses for your particular mental background music? Do you recognize these words of won't power:

It's too hard.
It's boring.
I can't do it.
I can't be bothered to diet today (my personal favorite).
I hate eating diet food.
I feel so deprived.
I can't bear to be hungry.
It's not worth it.
The weight is not coming off quickly enough.
I may as well give up.
I am too weak-willed.

I can't resist (insert favorite food here).
I've always failed before, I can *never* succeed.
Food is my only real comfort.
I work so hard, I need to treat myself.
I can't face another day of dieting.
I can't keep this healthy eating going.
I have no self-control.
I have to eat to deal with my stress.
I'm too busy right now.
Life's too short for all this deprivation.
I've just eaten that fudge cake so there's no point in dieting today.
I'll start again tomorrow.

Are there any other won't power thoughts that are personal to you? It's good to make a note of what your mind tells you. That way, you'll be able to get the upper hand. If you've never stopped to listen carefully to these thoughts, now would be a good time to start. Know what negative, self-defeating thoughts your mind is feeding you.

YOUR THOUGHTS ARE ENTIRELY SUBJECTIVE

There is a saying worth considering: "What you *think* is not necessarily true or real." Just because you think something doesn't make it scientifically provable. It is only your unique take on the subject. It's your mind's opinion based on all the evidence you keep inside you. This internal evidence is made up of everything that ever happened to you. Your mind's job is to collate all the evidence and make sense of it, to build up a picture of who you are and how you live your life.

These phrases of won't power are only the considered opinions of your mind, based on what has happened in the past. Therefore, when you hear, "I can't do it," it could be a reminder of past times when losing weight was just too hard and you gave up. There may have been many good reasons why you gave up, but your mind takes this sound bite as your personal truth and then feeds it back to you.

I like to listen to what my mind tries to tell me. It gives me a fascinating insight into the way the subconscious and conscious minds work together. Here's an example taken from my personal archives:

I decide that I'm going to lose some weight and I'm planning to start tomorrow. I'm confident I can do it. I have a plan. I feel fired up and ready to go.

My mind says these things to me: "But it's so hard to lose weight at your age." "I doubt you'll lose that much weight before you give up." "Remember that time when you did the ***** diet, you actually *put on* weight." "Why don't you put this off until summer?" "Diets don't work for you, they never have." "You'll have to start back at the gym, you know you hate that."

You have to admire the mind for its inventiveness. It seems to have an inexhaustible supply of won't power to make us want to give up.

What, therefore, might be the purpose of won't power? Why does the mind keep trying to defeat all the good intentions, particularly when it's obvious that losing weight and getting more healthy would be a good thing? While it may seem contradictory, your mind is trying to protect you. Its role is to keep you safe and prevent you from harm. It only has access to the data inside, the evidence from your past, it doesn't have the full objective picture. It makes decisions based on what seems the best course at the time.

If trying to lose weight in the past has made you miserable, hungry, tired, left out and downright grumpy, it's logical that your mind is going to try and put you off doing it again. But remember, just because you *think* something doesn't necessarily make it true or real. These won't power thoughts are only made of words and energy. You can easily challenge them. You can call them out.

YOU ALREADY HAVE WILLPOWER IN YOUR LIFE

One way to challenge all this negative thinking is to focus on another area of your life where you have total confidence and amazing willpower. A part of your life that is successful. I wonder if you can think of three specific areas of your life that fit this description. Small things or bigger things, it doesn't matter.

Keeping it nice and simple:

- What is your finest quality as a person?
- What is your best achievement?
- Think of a time when you succeeded against the odds.
- What part of your face or body do you like best?
- What skill do you possess that you are most proud of?

Indulge yourself and allow your mind to experience all the energy, confidence and inner strength that you feel when you think about these areas of your life. It's okay to keep reminding yourself about your good qualities, your achievements and successes.

Willpower, you see, is a skill or quality that you already possess. It can be developed, built upon and transferred to other areas of your life. Your mind can be trained to talk to you in the language of willpower. It can unlearn the habits of feeding you thoughts and ideas that are designed to defeat you and put you off creating that slim, healthy body you wish for.

This guided meditation, *Iron Willpower*, has been specifically designed to do just that, to reverse the negative, self-defeating thoughts of won't power and install all the positive, life-affirming thoughts of willpower. Using the track will change your inner dialogue over time so you receive increasing numbers of positive messages that are supportive of your journey towards a slim, healthy body.

If you have any doubts that this is possible, just remind yourself that all the won't power thoughts you now listen to (and believe are part of your true personality) got into your mind somehow. *You were not born thinking this way.* You learned how to do it from all your experiences in the past. It's totally possible to unlearn everything you think right now.

WHAT DOES WILLPOWER FEELS LIKE?

This guided meditation is deliberately short and concise. It's designed to be used frequently as a burst of inner strength to support you and keep you on track. It's easy to fit into your day. Like all guided meditations, the effects build up, growing more powerful every time you practice. Inner willpower also comprises mental and emotional energy that is tangible, giving you a real feeling inside. It will seem as if you have an immutable core of strength that will never weaken.

Once you have built up your willpower, you can use it to power other areas of your life. You can have control of it, using your willpower where it's needed. It will not interfere with parts of your life where you want to have soft, yielding qualities, where you wish to be flexible, magnanimous or show your vulnerable side. Having iron willpower will not change your personality. That is because you will always be in control. You will always be able to choose how to think and act.

If you are the type of person who values choice and independence, it's important to be reassured about this level of personal control you will still have. However, when your willpower is fully developed, you will have more choices at your disposal, choices that will make you strong and tough in the face of adversity.

DEVELOPING IRON WILLPOWER

Where does willpower come from and what will it feel like? Is it only about the thoughts in your head or is there more to it? Willpower comes from a center of energy called your "personal power spot" or, in Eastern philosophy, the solar plexus chakra, an energy center located right in your core. Called manipura, it is the center of personal power, characterized by these qualities:

- Willpower.
- Taking responsibility for one's life.
- Mental abilities and intellect.
- Personal opinions and beliefs.
- Making decisions, setting the direction.
- Clarity of judgments.
- Personal identity.
- Self-assurance.
- Self-discipline.
- Independence.

If this chakra could speak it would say: "Radiate your power into the world." When this energy center is glowing with light and full of power, you feel on top of the world, confident about your life's direction and your ability to realize your goals. You can imagine this chakra to be like a bright yellow sunflower with petals open to the sun. Use this mental picture to inspire your internal imaginings when you listen to the *Iron Willpower* track.

When you use the track, you'll be invited to build up the furnace of personal energy inside your solar plexus chakra. You will then be prompted to consider the six elements of willpower which are personal skills that you can focus on and energize. We break the concept of willpower down into six achievable and easily identifiable parts:

1. *Determination:* You are completely determined to lose all of your excess weight. Your mind is made up; you are fixed on your goal.

2. *Motivation:* The energy of your incentive to be slim and healthy, to love yourself and your life. You can see yourself in your slim future and it inspires you.
3. *Confidence:* You trust your abilities, you feel self-assured, you can do it!
4. *Focus:* You have total clarity about your goal. All your attention, your energy and your resources are concentrated on becoming slim and healthy.
5. *Tenacity:* Stubborn and persistent, you stick to your goal, never giving up, no matter what difficulties come your way.
6. *Mental toughness:* You've made up your mind and that is it! Mentally resolute and intractable, strong and resilient, you hold firmly on to your goal, despite all the distractions and temptations. The mind repels unwanted thoughts or ideas that might interfere with success.

You then proceed to energize these willpower skills and absorb them into your personal power spot which is your solar plexus chakra. It's beneficial to work with the mental symbol of a bright yellow sunflower and then build on it. Mental imagery that is clear and positive will give your mind a picture to work with that encapsulates all the positive messages you want to absorb deep inside yourself.

Hemi-Sync® frequencies have been designed to accompany each track, leading your mind into powerful, resourceful states where learning can be accelerated and change can be successfully accomplished. Your awareness will be receptive, open and expanded to absorb the messages, ideas, images and wisdom that will build up and reinforce your sense of iron willpower.

YOUR IMAGINATION IS A POWERFUL RESOURCE
You might wonder how something that you have only imagined can become your reality. Be in no doubt, your ability to imagine is a powerful resource, mostly underused, that can add creative force to

the inner messages you are now learning. At the heart of this idea is the perception that the subconscious mind does not easily distinguish between imagined and remembered material, as long as the imagined material is compelling, bright, enticing and believable. While imagination is accepted and revered for creative people, artists, writers, musicians, and children, as people grow into adulthood there is a tendency to dismiss imagined material as having less value than factual material. We are discouraged from using our imaginative skills. The adult world likes facts and science.

An interesting example of the successful use of imagination comes from the world of professional sport. Sports performance coaches use imagination, visualization and mental rehearsal in their work with professional athletes to enhance and perfect their sporting skills and competitive performance. Visualizing success appears to produce the same mental instructions to the body as real life actions. It has been found that mental imagery affects many cognitive processes in the brain including muscle control, awareness, preparation, and memory. When you engage in inner visualization, the brain is training itself for actual real-life performance. Your mind will be able to remember your visualization as if it was real and has already happened. Your body will also respond positively to your imaginings.

This idea is central to many of the guided meditations in this album. Therefore, feel empowered by what your mind is capable of. Decide to use your inner creative skills to the maximum of your abilities.

THE LANGUAGE OF WILLPOWER: AFFIRMATIONS
When you embrace iron willpower you'll not only have that fiery energy burning inside you that transforms into a strong rod of iron, reminding you of your unbreakable resolve. You'll also be listening to the new soundtrack of your mind speaking the words of willpower. These words and phrases will pop into your head and surprise you with their positivity. Your mind might choose to repeat some of the

affirmations that are embedded within the tracks. Or you may hear your inner voice speaking supportive phrases that are relevant to your unique circumstances. When you speak with the inner language of willpower, you *will* succeed. Every part of you, mind, body and spirit, will be determined, motivated, confident, focused, tenacious and filled with mental toughness.

I've listed below the affirmations on the track which speak the language of willpower. You can think about how each phrase sounds to you. Perhaps you prefer to change some of the phrases by using different words that have more meaning for you. You are in charge of how you want your new-found willpower to sound.

Using the affirmations as inspiration, write down 10 super-positive willpower phrases that are specific to your life. Or take 10 of the affirmations as your most important sayings. Be prepared for these phrases to become your new inner dialogue, and for you to respond positively to the way your mind will speak to you.

AFFIRMATIONS

I am determined to slim down to my goal weight.
Nothing is going to stop me. I am confident and focused.
I have iron willpower; I will succeed.
Food is delicious fuel for my body and mind.
I love to plan my meals for maximum enjoyment.
I enjoy giving myself good food to eat — in just the right amounts.
My stomach is about the size of a large orange.
That's the right amount of food for me to eat.
I only eat at mealtimes so I can appreciate my food.
I eat less but enjoy it more. I never feel deprived.
I listen to my body and pay attention to its messages.
I always give myself enough time to enjoy my food properly.
My food tastes great when I concentrate fully on what I'm eating.
I choose to be peaceful and quiet when I'm eating.

At the end of each meal I feel full and satisfied.

I make every meal a special occasion.

I make getting slim my top priority.

My health and vitality is important, to me and those I care about.

I know I can succeed if I eat well and stick to my plan.

I feel full of energy and radiate good health.

Every morning I feel slimmer and healthier.

I look forward each day, enjoying my food and feeling slimmer.

Being organized is my way to ensure success.

I look forward to seeing my slimmer body revealing itself.

I look forward to the time in between meals which are my favorite times of day.

Every day I can enrich my life with new exciting things to do.

Exercise is my way of making myself feel fitter and stronger.

I enjoy trying new things, new activities that make me feel alive.

When I try something new, I feel my confidence grow.

My body appreciates all the attention I give it.

When I'm active, I am raising my metabolism.

When I eat out, I feel completely in control.

I make wise choices when I eat out and enjoy myself fully.

Eating out is all about the occasion and having fun.

I include my temptation foods in my meals so I can enjoy them in moderation.

Food no longer has power over me.

My favorite foods are enjoyable in small amounts.

I am polite when others try to make me eat more.

I prefer to have a meal that is moderate, rather than overloaded.

In social situations, I feel no pressure to overeat.

I smile and continue to eat less but enjoy it more.

I choose relaxation to deal with life's everyday pressures.

I no longer use food to cope with stressful situations.

Things that used to bother me in the past no longer have the power to hurt me.

I face challenges head on, calm and relaxed no matter what happens.

People and situations that hinder me — I just let go of them.
Everybody notices how much more happy and confident I am.
I deserve to be slim because I work hard at it.
I send myself regular messages of support.
I give myself praise every day for the good job I'm doing.
I reinforce my value with regular compliments.
When I stumble, I pick myself right up.
Life's ups and downs teach me how to be strong and determined.
I like and respect myself, inside and out.
I am worthy of love and attention.
I allow my inner self to shine.
Life is good and I feel great.
As I reveal my slim, healthy body I grow in confidence.
I look forward to my slim, healthy future.
Every step I take will guide me there.

These affirmations appear in many of the tracks because this regular, positive reinforcement will be crucial to your success. It's not possible to create a slim, healthy body while your inner dialogue with yourself is relentlessly negative. However, you don't have to consciously do anything to change your self-talk. This program will embed positive thinking deep inside you as you practice with the tracks.

It's interesting to be aware of your thoughts and the quality of your inner dialogue. As you open yourself up to the positive words of willpower you will absorb an amazing new language. Soon you'll hear your mind talking to you using these positive messages as inspiration. It will sound really lovely.

CHAPTER 4
CRAVING CONTROL

CRAVINGS ARE LINKED WITH MEMORIES

The relationship with food begins at birth. It is a deep and complex relationship that is intermingled with all of the human emotions it's possible to imagine. People connect food with the experiences they have either enjoyed or endured (and all the different nuances of emotion in between) during their lifetimes. The senses add an extra dimension to the memories.

Therefore tastes, smells, feelings, sights and sounds all shape the quality of memories that make up a person's life story. Pause for a moment and get a sense of how rich and varied your own memories are, simply due to the way you have stored them with all the unique extra layers of meaning from your senses and your emotions. How beautiful it is to be able to think about a happy food memory and, by getting quiet and focusing inside, you can almost step inside the memory, reliving each moment and re-experiencing the pleasure.

If there were only happy memories to revisit, life might be a lot easier. It follows that you may also have food memories that are connected with other, less positive emotions. Any negative or unhappy food memories that are stored inside your mind will also have the power to influence thoughts, behaviors and emotions in the present day.

WHAT ARE YOUR CRAVING FOODS?

Consider for a moment what foods you most rely on in your life, foods that you would struggle to stop eating. Are these the foods you *need* to eat? Or that you can't resist? Are these diet-breaking foods?

Sweet or savory, bland or strong-tasting, craving foods are very personal. These foods are doing something extra for you in your life, adding another dimension to your eating experience. You might associate your craving food with a feeling of comfort, of safety, of things in your life being made better. The food may remind you of happier times. During your childhood years you may have eaten your craving food as a treat or a reward or to take your mind off a scraped knee. It will be interesting to discover what memories and emotions are linked to your own craving foods.

Some popular examples:
- Freshly baked bread with butter on it. Fresh bread is a renowned diet-breaking food.
- Chocolate, that popular remedy for everything horrible that happens in life.
- Cheese in all its forms: on a cracker, in a sandwich, melting on a pizza or adorning a bowl of pasta.

- Apple pie and whipped cream might be your downfall.
- Spicy food can be irresistible.
- A gooey cinnamon roll with vanilla frosting.
- Potato chips in all the popular flavors have ruined so many weight loss plans.

Try and identify five foods that you cannot resist. Your personal diet-breaking foods. It's not necessary to recall the memories or emotions you associate with these foods. That information is for your mind to know and ultimately for your mind to release.

If craving a particular food or foods is stopping you from losing all your unwanted weight and achieving that slim, healthy body you wish for, now is the time to dissolve the emotional links between the craving foods and those memories. This *Craving Control* track is specifically designed to achieve this.

INTRODUCING ACUTAPPING TO RELEASE EMOTIONS

The track introduces an effective treatment which is generically called acutapping. It has many forms in complementary therapy, traceable to its roots in Chinese medicine. You may already be familiar with acupuncture, shiatsu and reflexology, all of which are known as energy therapies. Acutapping is non-invasive energy therapy and it can be applied by a therapist or it can be self-applied. As a powerful self-help technique, it has many uses.

The most significant beneficial use of acutapping, as it's applied in modern complementary therapy, is its effectiveness in neutralizing and releasing *negative* emotions and thoughts. You can use simple and easy-to-apply acutapping techniques to let go of negative thoughts, emotions, ideas, beliefs and behaviors. When tapping along to simple therapeutic words, your mind is instructed to let go of unwanted emotions that act as fuel for your cravings.

Furthermore, acutapping makes a harmonious therapy partner to all kinds of guided meditation work. When you listen to guided meditations, the messages tend to be positive ones. You absorb positive ways of thinking and feeling as you listen. Now add into that mix some acutapping therapy which focuses on releasing negative thoughts and emotions. If you want to change your life in a positive way it makes sense to work on neutralizing those negative thoughts and feelings that may be blocking your progress. As you add more of the positive and you let go of more of the negative there can be a seismic shift of attitude inside.

At the end of this chapter, there are suggestions for further exploration of energy therapy. As a passionate advocate for these techniques, I have witnessed first-hand the life-changing results that can be achieved. This craving control procedure will provide an introduction to all the many forms of energy therapy that are available and make you inquisitive for more.

The verbally-guided meditation will take you through the stages of a simplified acutapping sequence with words that are intended to target the emotional tug associated with craving foods. The acutapping sequence is therefore designed for the purpose of craving control. However, once you have learned this simple technique, you can expand your understanding and discover other acutapping techniques that you can utilize in your daily life.

There is a saying that has become associated with energy therapy: "Try it on everything." "Everything" can mean physical illness, pain and discomfort, psychological issues and all manner of emotional distress. Most everyday problems have an emotional aspect to them, either as a causal factor or as a consequence. When you work on releasing the emotions, many unexpected benefits can result. We therefore always keep an open mind when using energy therapies.

LOCATING THE TAPPING POINTS

Before you begin the track, you need to identify the meridian points and practice tapping on them. The description of the points is written below. The images that follow will also help you to locate these points.

Finding the eight points (can be on either side of the body):

1. *Eyebrow point*: the beginning of your eyebrow on either side. Feel your eyebrow under your finger. Tap 10 times with your middle finger. (Fig. 1)
2. *Side eye point*: about a finger width from the side of your eye. Tap 10 times with your middle finger. (Fig. 1)
3. *Under eye point*: directly under your iris, feel the eye socket bone under your finger, tap firmly but carefully. Tap 10 times with your middle finger. (Fig. 1)
4. *Under nose point*: between your nose and your upper lip. Tap 10 times with your middle finger. (Fig. 1)
5. *Collarbone point*: you feel for your collarbone, then move down about two inches. It's the flat area of your breastbone. Tap it 10 times with three or four fingers. (Fig. 2)
6. *Index finger point*: located on either index finger on the nail bed. Hold your hand out horizontally in front of you, thumb pointing towards your chest. You see the side of your index finger. The nail bed you can see is the tapping point. Use your other index finger and firmly tap 10 times on this point. (Fig. 3)
7. *Little finger point*: located on either little finger on the nail bed. Hold your hand out horizontally in front of you, thumb pointing towards your chest. You see the side of your little finger. The nail bed you can see is the tapping point. Use your other index finger and firmly tap 10 times on this point. (Fig. 3)
8. *Palm of hand point*: press your thumb into the center of your palm, supporting your hand gently with your fingers at the back of your hand. Squeeze your thumb into your palm. (Fig. 4)

Figure 1: The eyebrow point, the side eye point, the under eye point and the under nose point.

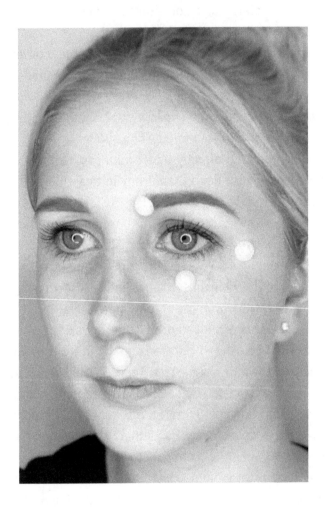

Figure 2: The collarbone points.

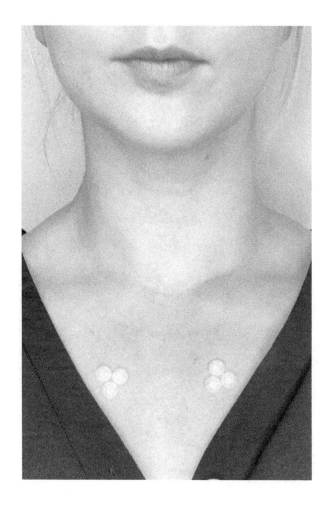

Figure 3: The index finger point and the little finger point.

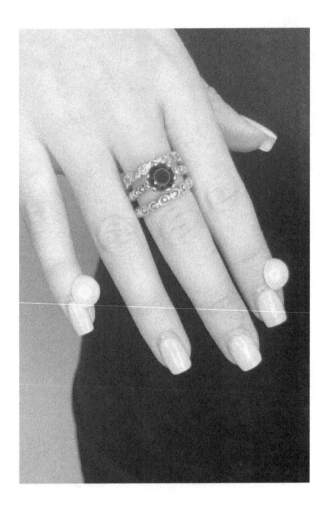

Figure 4: The palm of hand point.

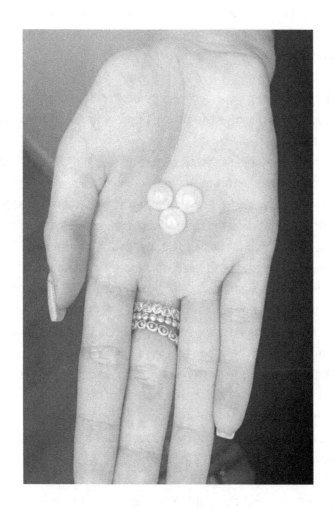

THE CRAVING CONTROL EXERCISE:

Start by taking a deep breath to center yourself. Pick up a food. Have a good look at it. Smell it. Sense the essence of the food. Then when you are ready, have a taste.

Take a moment to allow your mind and emotions to make the subconscious link, but keep yourself *focused on the food*. Put the food down and ready yourself for some energy work.

1. Begin tapping your *eyebrow point*, and repeat these words as you tap: "I dissolve the threads that bind me to this food. I am set free."
2. Now to the *side eye point*, tap it and say: "I dissolve the threads that bind me to this food. I am set free."
3. Now to the *under eye point*, tap it and say: "I dissolve the threads that bind me to this food. I am set free."
4. Now to the *under nose point*, tap the point and say: "I dissolve the threads that bind me to this food. I am set free."
5. Now to the *collarbone point*, tap with 3 or 4 fingers and say: "I dissolve the threads that bind me to this food. I am set free."
6. Now to the *index finger point*. Tap and say: "I dissolve the threads that bind me to this food. I am set free."
7. Now to the *little finger point*. Tap and say: "I dissolve the threads that bind me to this food. I am set free."
8. Finally, take hold of your hand, and press the *center of your palm* with your thumb and say: "I dissolve the threads that bind me to this food. I am set free."

Breathe slowly in and then out. You are sending a message to your emotions to balance all your thoughts and feelings about this food.

Now pick up the food again and smell it, taste it and notice any differences in your responses to this food. Notice also the way your emotions respond to this food. Then when you are ready, go through the acutapping procedure again. You will be guided to do so by the verbal instructions in the track.

You carry out the craving control exercise in the waking state. You assemble your craving foods in small amounts. Work on one at a time, until you have done sufficient tapping, as prompted during the track, to dissolve the emotional links between you and the food.

TAPPING HINTS

Tap with the pad of your middle finger, except on your collarbone point where you can tap with three or four fingers; it's a big point. The tapping action is like using a tiny silver hammer to tap in a tiny nail. If you feel any tenderness when you tap the points, this will fade with practice.

Make sure you feel it. You are making an energy intervention in the energy meridians under your skin.

Tap each point about 10 times. This is a flexible number, but generally continue to tap during the time it takes you to say the words.

Tap the two finger points, the index finger point and the little finger point, using the index finger of your other hand. Tap on the nail bed slightly towards you, hold your little finger stiff while you tap. You will soon be able to get into a comfortable rhythm.

You can tap on either side of the body, the meridians are located symmetrically on each side. When you tap on one meridian, the energy change radiates throughout your own system and affects your energy system all over your body.

Imagine as you tap that the energy is being released from inside you when you lift your finger *away* from the tapping point.

Practice makes perfect. Look in the mirror from time to time and check you are tapping on the right spots. You'll soon get into a rhythm. More is better. Do it over and over for 10 minutes and sense how that feels.

When you start, it may feel as if nothing is happening. As you practice more, your energy meridians will respond and become more receptive to the acutapping work.

Intention is very important in energy work. As you tap you send a strong message to your inner self that you want to release all the emotions connected with the food.

THE MEANING OF THE ACUTAPPING POINTS

Energy meridians, according to traditional Chinese medicine, have names associated with their location and meaning within the body. Points on the energy meridians are associated with physical health issues and also psychological/emotional issues. It is only possible here to give a very general perspective about this subject. Words that we use in our western culture may not equate accurately to traditional Chinese medicine. Nevertheless, it's helpful to have some insight into this fascinating area of complementary therapy. For balance, I have chosen to include tapping points from each of the five elements:

- Water
- Wood
- Fire
- Earth
- Metal

The *eyebrow point* is the second point on the bladder meridian (water element). It can be associated with fear and anxiety, oversensitivity, phobias, stress and worry. When balanced, it is associated with willpower and courage. (Inner Direction).

The *side eye point* is the beginning point on the gallbladder meridian (wood element). It can be associated with anger, upset, impatience, resentment and disappointment. There is a link with a competitive spirit and being a high achiever. When balanced, it is associated with good humor. (Harmony).

The *under eye point* is the beginning of the stomach meridian (earth element) associated with anxiety, feelings of being burdened, frustration and compensatory eating. It may be linked with feeling unsatisfied. When balanced, it promotes the feeling of being calm and satisfied. (Contentment).

The *under nose point* is on the conception vessel, one of the main energy circulation vessels for the body. When tapped, the conception vessel promotes increased energy circulation and may be associated with feeling more energetic and having more zest for living.

The *collarbone point* is the beginning of the kidney meridian (water element) and may be associated with anxiety, lack of personal drive and lack of courage. When balanced, it links to feelings of courage, confidence and personal drive (which we might call *willpower*). (Gentle spirit).

The *index finger point* is point 1 on the large intestine meridian (metal element). It can be associated with grief, obstructions and difficulty with letting go of things. When tapped, it promotes positive thinking and letting go. (Letting go).

The *little finger point* is located at the end of heart meridian (fire element). It can be associated with emotional trauma, hyper-sensitivity, restlessness and being overactive. When balanced, this point opens up consciousness and develops unconditional love, compassion and joyfulness. (Unconditional love).

The *center of palm point* is on the heart governor meridian and acts like a hotline to deep heart protection energy, to early memories, sometimes even as far back as birth. Heart protection is vital for our balanced emotions so the acutapping sequence finishes with this point. You hold your hand and press your thumb into your palm.

CRAVING CONTROL VERSUS ENJOYMENT

Once you have learned this simple acutapping sequence, you can use it to dissolve those emotional links or "threads that bind you" (in your mind) to the food. When you are practicing, you may notice the food does not smell the same when you are holding it to your nose. If you taste it, it may not seem as appetizing. People often report the acutapping sequence makes the food lose its appeal. However, do not worry. This acutapping procedure will not stop you enjoying your favorite foods in the future. All that happens is the foods will no longer have the same power over you. You will be able to choose whether to enjoy them or not. The food will no longer have the power to break your self control or ruin your diet.

You may need to practice several times to get all those emotional threads dissolved. Every time you practice energy therapies, you send a powerful signal to your subconscious mind that you intend to change. It also follows that your relationship with the foods you love will no longer be based on emotions about things that happened in the past.

ACUTAPPING ADAPTED FOR OTHER SITUATIONS

You can adapt this acutapping procedure for any problems that you may encounter, either in connection with becoming slimmer and healthier or in any area of your life. All you do is adapt the words, the tapping remains the same. Formulate what you want to work on into words that reflect how you think and feel. The following examples will give you a template to guide you while you design you own phrases.

- I release the fear that I'll fail at this weight loss journey. I am full of courage.
- I transform my habit of snacking in the afternoon. I enjoy being in control.
- I let go of pressure to eat at family parties. I am my own person.
- I change my attitude to what gives me enjoyment. Life is full of possibilities.
- I cocoon myself against people who get me down. I am safe and protected.

Note that your words will be the right words. You will automatically express your thoughts and feelings in the language you naturally use. Inspiration for more ideas about words to use to express won't power and the words for positive affirmations can be found through-out this book.

IF YOU WANT TO FIND OUT MORE

This simplified version of acutapping can serve as a great introduction to the full experience of energy therapy. Across the world, there are energy therapists who are spreading the word and teaching ind-ividuals these techniques that will then help them to overcome emotional problems, psychological problems, self-defeating patterns of behavior and blocks to success. This is an innovative and growing area of personal development.

Once you have learned one of the many popular acutapping pro-cedures, and you are able to work effectively on your own, there is potential to let go of a host of negative thoughts, emotions and behaviors that may be holding you back. It will take practice, time and dedication but the results will far outweigh the energy you put in. It is always recommended to work with a professional therapist if you have any problems that may require one-to-one treatment. As with all complementary therapies, they complement the diagnosis and treatment from your medical professional. They are not a substitute for medical treatment.

If you are interested in finding out more, consult the internet to find professional organizations in your location, accredited teachers and trainers who can instruct you to learn how to fully utilize such techniques for your own wellbeing. While there are many excellent books, videos and articles available, it is highly recommended to learn, in the first instance, from a professional energy therapist. Books cannot give you the same initial experience of energy change that a qualified and experienced professional can.

Check the *Resources for Further Work* section at the end of this book for ideas on how to learn more about energy therapies.

CHAPTER 5
METABOLISM BOOST

The metabolism boost track utilizes a creative approach to changing the rate you use energy for all your basic functions. Boosting your metabolism will help you access more energy and create the slim, healthy body you wish for. Guided meditations make use of your imagination, your powers of visualization and your ability to engage in mental rehearsal. These same mental techniques are also extensively used to enhance sports performance. There is increasing evidence from top athletes that mental training can help take sports performance to the next level. From basketball players to Olympic athletes to golfers and tennis players, the inner work done using mental rehearsal is considered by athletes and their coaches to be as important as physical training to ensure peak performance. You can therefore have confidence you'll be able to boost your metabolism using your own inner powers of imagination, visualization and mental rehearsal.

HOW IS IT POSSIBLE TO INFLUENCE YOUR METABOLISM?
You might think your metabolic rate is pre-set. However, it is already influenced by your daily activity levels, the kinds of foods you eat, the temperature of your environment and how much mental activity you

engage in. Metabolic rate is also subject to influences from the past which can include over-strict dieting or times in your life when your activity levels were low. Because your metabolic rate is *already* influenced by so many factors, it is possible to issue direct commands to boost your own, individual rate of energy burn.

You might have doubts about whether it's possible to have control over your metabolism, or any other aspect of your life that seems to be outside of your conscious control. However, far from being *uncontrolled*, the level of control that is exercised inside your body to keep you healthy is truly amazing. The body/mind system is a finely-tuned organic machine, with sophisticated controls in place for every function required to keep you alive. Your body/mind system is always monitoring influences from your environment, both externally and internally. Adjustments are constantly being made inside to ensure "homeostasis" or internal balance, to put it simply. You might imagine your body/mind system is always listening and learning, making adjustments and balancing everything inside you. Therefore, during this track, if you make your instructions clear, unambiguous and believable, the message will be heard. It will be absorbed into your subconscious mind to exert a powerful influence over the way your whole body works.

As already mentioned earlier, sports performance coaches ensure athletes use all their senses to make the mental rehearsal of their sports discipline as realistic as possible. It seems the body responds by acting "as if" the experience was real. Imagination also allows you to rehearse only *positive* outcomes, thereby conditioning the mind and body for success.

In everyday life, the human mind will often revert to negative thinking, preferring to dwell on failures and over-thinking problems when things do not go according to plan. By imagining, visualizing and rehearsing *positive* outcomes you can counteract this natural human characteristic. With the scene now set, you can go inside yourself when you use this track and work directly on your metabolism, instructing it clearly and unequivocally to work harder, release more energy for you to use and help you feel full of vitality.

BASE METABOLIC RATE

Everyone has a base metabolic rate. It's possible to calculate your own metabolic rate from many tools that are available on the internet. Of course, these calculations are based on population averages and adjusted for a person's age, gender, height and weight and lifestyle, thus making the resulting number an approximation, not an exact figure.

It's estimated that anywhere between 50 to 80% of the energy you need to live is used up by your body to carry out all the basic functions to keep you alive. When scientists test base metabolic rate in the laboratory, the subject must be situated in a controlled temperature environment, in a resting position and not in the process of digesting food (which uses up extra energy). It's fascinating to note that a considerable amount of your total energy is used up in keeping your body at the right temperature. Therefore, when all your internal energy requirements are factored in, this leaves between 20 to 50% remaining for all the other activities in your life. This might include wriggling in your sleep, sneezing, digesting your meals or running to catch a bus. You might be using up your energy by enduring a brutal two-hour gym session or you may be conserving energy by lying on the sofa pointing the remote control at the TV. Everything uses energy. When you think about how energetic your waking activities are, it's amazing that the majority of your energy is used simply keeping you alive and functioning at about 98 degrees Fahrenheit.

Many people experience days when they feel they have no energy, no spark, when it's a struggle to find the energy to keep going until bedtime. Conversely, there will be days when you are aware your body is buzzing with energy and you can do more physical activity than you would normally do. You may associate not having enough energy with being on a weight loss diet. Feeling tired and sluggish can make you want to eat calorific foods to feel more energetic. It's important, therefore, to work at boosting your energy levels so you avoid giving in to temptation and overeating.

During this track you will focus inside to visualize your personal metabolic rate, allowing your subconscious awareness to share this information with you. You will then instruct your internal systems to boost your energy output so you can use more energy and make your metabolism work for you. When you feel energetic, your journey towards your slim, healthy body will be easy and enjoyable.

IMAGINING YOUR INNER THERMOSTAT

In this track, we focus on the inner thermostat, a simple image or symbol for the mind to lock into. Working to boost the reading on that thermostat sends a strong message to your inner control systems. The message you send is that you intend to use more energy in your daily life. Maybe your body has got into the habit of sending the energy from the food you eat for storage which manifests as extra pounds around your middle. If this is the case, there will not be an abundance of available energy for you to use for your everyday activities.

You can send a new message to your body/mind system about your personal equation between energy release and energy storage. This track contains the instructions to use your energy up, make the food you eat work hard for you and, by doing so, send more energy into all parts of your body for maximum aliveness.

Within each cell are several cell structures called the mitochondria. These are the energy sources for cell metabolism. Replicated in the cells throughout the body, the job of cell mitochondria is to turn fuel from food and oxygen from breathing into the energy that powers every part of you. Energy is released to carry out vital cell activities and to contribute to the healthy functioning of your body. We can imagine that the mitochondria are the "furnaces" inside each cell. For your own mental image, you can think of these cell structures as brightly colored elongated ovals, floating around inside each of your cells, functioning as powerhouses of energy production.

By visualizing these important cell structures when you listen to this track, you send a strong message to turn up the thermostat in each tiny furnace. You want to use your available energy more freely, so you can feel it glowing inside you. This image of cell mitochondria can be your inspiration when using the track.

Once you have turned up your thermostat and commanded the cell mitochondria to burn more fuel, it's useful to focus inside and have an enhanced awareness of the energy produced by your body. The track encourages you to be aware of this as an energy wave inside you.

By practicing this inner work, your mind and body will have clear instructions from you to boost your metabolism. If there has been any doubt in the past, if your inner thermostat has been slowed down by factors including your diet or lifestyle or health issues, you now have the opportunity to send yourself a "metabolism boost" message which is loud and clear.

ACTIVITY IS IMPORTANT

Your energy usage is also influenced by how physically active you are. While your base metabolic rate is all about energy used for basic functions which keep you alive, your activity levels account for the remaining 20-50% of your total energy use. Everything you do, as mentioned before, from sleeping, to showering, to eating, sitting at your computer or shouting at the neighbor's dog, every physical activity you engage in will influence your metabolism in a positive way. You are therefore encouraged to develop a passion for activity and to take part in activities that boost your heart and strengthen your muscles. All kinds of activity will raise your energy usage. Make up your mind to be more active in any way you can.

Your mind also uses a considerable amount of energy. When your mind is active, creative and full of inspiration, it will burn more energy than if you are passive and can't be bothered to take on new mental challenges. Seeking out activities that are mentally stimulating will also boost your mood and make you feel fulfilled. Aim high. Consider a new activity that will really challenge you.

Use this track regularly. It has been kept deliberately short and concise to fit in around any schedule. Challenge yourself to boost your own metabolic rate to a higher figure. Be curious about how much of a positive boost you can gain by doing this. Notice how much more energy you have in your everyday life. Feel pleased and satisfied with your achievement, then use your energy to get even more active.

CHAPTER 6
SLIM WHILE YOU SLEEP

"This track, *Slim While You Sleep,* incorporates powerful mind programming. Before you listen, you must read and fully understand the accompanying instructions. Sleeping is your time of relaxation, restoration and resourcefulness. During sleep, your mind can reset itself to a more positive way of thinking so that, when you wake, you will be clear headed, refreshed and full of positive resolve."

— *Slim While You Sleep,* Track 6

It is important for you to understand this track fully prior to using it. That is because the track is a software program for your mind. It has a specific function. While you can understand the track by listening to it, you will fully understand it and know how it works by reading this chapter, or by checking the summary in the booklet that comes with the album.

YOU CONTROL WHEN TO RUN THE PROGRAM

The bedtime command to run the subconscious program automatically during sleep is "SLIM WHILE YOU SLEEP." When you say or think these words at bedtime before you fall asleep, your mind will accept the command to run the program. It is important to understand that you have control of this subconscious program after you have installed it by listening to the track several times. It will only run when you command it. You will always be in control.

UNDERSTANDING HOW SUBCONSCIOUS PROGRAMS WORK

In Chapter 2, we explored the idea that our minds design and install subconscious programs to carry out everyday tasks that require more processing power than the conscious mind is capable of. That idea, the model of the conscious mind and subconscious mind is central to the operation of this track. Therefore, to revisit the definitions:

Conscious mind — awake and aware, has judgment, decision making capability, opinions and logical thought. It has a sense of what is right and wrong, good and bad. It likes to categorize things and make sense of them.

Subconscious mind — on duty 24 hours a day, the data repository, the location of your memories, software programs and belief system. The imagination exists in this part of the mind. Dreams are created here. The subconscious is benign in that it does not judge the data. It has no sense of right and wrong, good and bad. It organizes the data so the conscious mind can make sense of it.

Remember, this is a model, a simplified way of defining something very complex to make understanding easier.

Human minds have the natural capability to write their own software (or subconscious programs). The examples I gave earlier were learning to walk and learning to drive a car. Even something as mundane as cleaning your teeth offers a fascinating insight into how the mind writes programs to carry out complex activities and make them seem simple. When you break "teeth cleaning" down into individual actions, you end up with a sequence of muscle movements involving the tensing and relaxing of your arm muscles, your grip on the toothbrush, the changing direction of movement around your teeth, the sensing of when you have cleaned each section and when to move on to the next, the control of your salivary flow, the foam, the spitting and so on. All ending up with a good rinse.

Each tiny element is intricate, requiring a sophisticated program to make it happen. Yet you can do it without thinking. Next time you clean your teeth, be aware of exactly how complex this small part of your everyday life is. And be aware of what is making it happen. You may even be doing something else while you are cleaning your teeth, such as planning a new bathroom, or worrying about work or listening to music or deciding how to fix that annoying dripping tap. Your sub-conscious mind has designed and installed a software program to make teeth cleaning happen for you. And while it does, your conscious mind can get on with its own list of jobs.

This understanding of the power of the subconscious mind carries the potential for you to take this innate ability you possess to the next level. You can install precise software which will support your journey towards a slim, healthy body, software that will run a program in your mind to clear the way for you to succeed. The software works by eliminating the mental blocks that may be holding you back.

THE PROGRAM WILL NEUTRALIZE NEGATIVE THOUGHTS
I come back to that diet wrecker called won't power, the mental blocks that stop you from getting to where you want to be. What if it were possible to install specific software to neutralize all that won't power that already exists inside you? If you could neutralize and dissolve all the negative self-talk, the way would be clear for you to power onwards towards a slim, healthy body. You would want to install this software program, wouldn't you? But first you would want to know exactly how it works, if it's appropriate for you to use, and if it comes with the right safety features. It's always good to check the small print before you sign up for something new.

Another way to describe the subconscious program in this track is to compare it with the kind of computer maintenance program you can run to clean up your hard drive or defragment your disk. I know only enough about computers to be able to function at a basic level, so my explanation may fall short if you are an expert in this field. However, from time to time, particularly with older computers which have less data storage space, you may be prompted to run a program that deletes old files, empties your recycle bin and reorganizes the remaining data into an orderly pattern, thus freeing up much needed disk space for you to use.

If you prefer a less computer-based explanation: cleaning out your hall cupboard of all the items you no longer use, putting everything back where it belongs, sorting important stuff into properly labeled boxes and freeing up some room for all the shiny new things you want to buy. The key message here is that there is *stuff to throw away*, and by throwing it away you will gain many benefits. That is an easy idea to understand when you are thinking about overcrowded cupboards, but not so easy when you think about de-cluttering your mind.

At the heart of this *Slim While You Sleep* track is the idea that your subconscious mind will respond to your instructions. If you command your subconscious mind to do something — and the command is clear, direct, literal and capable of being executed — the subconscious mind will have no choice but to implement your command. Simply because you don't know how to do this in your everyday waking life does not mean it can't be done.

This track commands your subconscious mind to search for and neutralize all the negative thoughts, mental blocks, unhelpful beliefs and obstructive behaviors that may prevent you from creating a slim, healthy body. Once all those pieces of mental mind clutter have been neutralized, they no longer have any power over you. You will be able to create your slim, healthy body with a clear mind.

MEDITATION AND SLEEP

This track is designed to be used at bedtime. The suggestions at the end encourage you to sink into restful sleep. Making sure you are fully ready for sleep, with all your bedtime routines carried out, will ensure you get the best results and the best sleep. If you listen through head-phones, you'll be prompted to remove them at the end of the track. There is nothing worse than drifting off the sleep only to be woken up by painful ears! The music continues for about 15 minutes after the end of the vocal guidance so you can drift off in your own time.

A general word about sleeping and guided meditations: it is perfectly natural to sink into sleep from time to time, even when the guidance is engaging and you are enjoying it. Sleep is always nearby when you experience mental relaxation. You may even feel as if you slip in and out of sleep when you listen, as if you zone out for a while then come back to hearing what is being said. "Music only" tracks encourage this sense of free mental travel, as there are no instructions about what to do or what to think.

When you get these feelings, you are experiencing what it is like to be free from conscious interference. Your waking, conscious mind has stepped out for a while, leaving you and your subconscious to enjoy each other's company. If you're ready for sleep you will drift into true sleep, which is when other changes happen. It's well known that during sleep your body is infused with special "sleeping" chemicals that keep you still and quiet and anaesthetized, instead of tossing and turning or enacting your dreams or walking in your sleep.

If you fall asleep during this or any of the tracks, your subconscious mind will still be listening, very carefully and very attentively. It has awareness for 24 hours a day. It's a common misconception that falling asleep makes the meditation less valid. However, you could also argue the important suggestions will be absorbed deep inside your mind with less conscious interference.

My clients were always telling me their meditation homework made them fall asleep. I told them, "That's because you are tired. Your mind will take out of the meditation what it most needs. Which often…is sleep." Therefore, take what comes to you with all of the tracks in this album that you practice when you are lying down or sitting in a relaxing chair. However, if you fall asleep during the *Craving Control Waking Meditation* — which is designed to be experienced while you're awake — you really do need more sleep!

SUMMARY OF THE TRACK

Begin by getting everything ready for sleep. Get really comfortable in bed. For the duration of the track you should always be lying flat in a symmetrical position with legs and hands uncrossed. This position helps prevent any physical discomfort from disturbing your focus.

The first section takes you on a relaxing journey, noticing various sensations around your body. You dissociate your mind from your body and focus on your inner feelings. There are pauses in the music while the Hemi-Sync® frequencies to do their special work. Then you clear a space in your mind. I often refer to this as your inner black-board, where you can look at images or write things or imagine things. In this case your mind simply needs to be open and receptive for the work ahead.

"I now call in your wise inner self to assist with this process. As you listen to these words, it will seem like to you are speaking directly to yourself."

— *Slim While You Sleep*, Track 6

Your wise inner self is a regular traveling companion during many tracks on this album. I think of this inner energy being as concerned with your earthly life, the challenges of your physical existence. This contrasts with a more familiar energy figure called your higher self, an energy being that's more focused on your spiritual life. Your wise inner self has the benefit of knowing everything that is part of you, everything that has made you who you are. It has access to your subconscious mind so it understands the many challenges you face. Its job is to provide down-to-earth guidance about your everyday life with all its attendant difficulties. It knows how hard life can sometimes be. It can empathize. It is your cheerleader on earth, always supporting you. Your wise inner self never speaks to you using that negative, self defeating mind chatter we all suffer from. It is wiser than that!

We ask your wise inner self to join us on this journey as a companion and supporter and to oversee the subconscious program you are going to install. You may imagine this wise being holding your hand or standing close by, supporting you. Now we address your subconscious mind directly, reminding you and your subconscious mind about all the positive, important functions it carries out for you.

"Subconscious mind, you keep me safe and protected, always doing the best for me. You store and maintain all the recorded memories of everything that has ever happened to me. You are the keeper of my memories. You organize everything into order of significance based on the emotional content — both positive and negative. Memories that have emotional importance, you keep them close so I can refer to them when I need to. That is how you keep me safe and protected, by reminding me about the difference between good experiences and experiences that might hurt me. You help me to know in advance what might hurt so that I can avoid it. You have constructed my belief system from all these recorded memories. I understand who I am and how I fit in this world."

— *Slim While You Sleep,* Track 6

Now you are ready to listen to the direct commands of this program. Your subconscious mind is very literal. It will understand your direct instructions. It doesn't respond positively to words like "less" or "more" or "some." It likes facts and numbers and certainty. Therefore the verbal commands will sound more akin to a series of orders rather than a soothing guided journey, and that is how it should be.

You hear the instructions as if you are speaking directly to yourself. You tell your subconscious mind that you intend to change. This has the effect of signaling your new intentions. Your subconscious mind will require confirmation that you are set on this journey towards a slim, healthy body, and that there may be challenges that take you out of your comfort zone. You tell your subconscious mind unequivocally, "I am ready to face those challenges."

> "Creating a slim, healthy body for life is now my goal. I instruct you therefore to integrate that goal as our primary objective. Creating a slim, healthy body for life becomes our goal. We will work together in a purposeful and cooperative way."
> — *Slim While You Sleep,* Track 6

The next section of the track introduces the command to your subconscious mind to search for and remove (with the assistance of your wise inner self) all negative thoughts, mental blocks, unhelpful beliefs and obstructive behaviors that are stopping you from achieving your goal of a slim, healthy body. Think of this like an internet search through all of your recorded memories.

When this search has been successfully concluded, the next command acts to neutralize the emotional energy connected with the negative thoughts, mental blocks, unhelpful beliefs and obstructive behaviors, making them powerless to affect you.

It is always important to be specific. That is why there are limits set in this mental clean-up process. I am confident that human minds keep all their recorded memories in an orderly fashion, with a proper filing system in place. There is unwanted negative mind clutter, but it is still stored in an orderly way so it can be accessed instantly whenever it's required. This orderly filing system allows this subconscious program to do its work efficiently in accordance with the instructions.

There next follows a command to the subconscious mind to design and install a program to clean up the recorded memories and to do it automatically during sleep.

"You will integrate this subconscious program into your normal sleep-time activity of organizing, sorting and filing all new memories that I record from my everyday experiences. As you cooperate with our wise inner self on which memories to keep and which to discard, you will automatically neutralize and dissolve all negative thoughts, mental blocks, unhelpful beliefs and obstructive behaviors as you encounter them."

— Slim While You Sleep, Track 6

There follows a list of potential negative thoughts, mental blocks, unhelpful beliefs and obstructive behaviors. These are the thoughts and sayings of won't power. They are set out in the first person, in a short form. Your mind will know them. If any of the words are not exactly as you would say them, your mind and your wise inner self will make adjustments. At the end of the list you instruct your subconscious mind to include such additional thoughts or sayings "that are personal to me because of my unique life experience."

It may seem that there is a long list of negative, unhelpful mental chatter that you have to listen to. You may hold the view that you should only ever express positive things, that you should always be positive about your life. The popular view of therapy is that it is invariably about *positive thinking*. However, I am more realistic about what the mind prefers to hold on to. I *know* that all the negative mental clutter in your mind is still there, waiting, brooding, stored in its filing cabinets, and it's ready to speak to you and frustrate your heartfelt wishes about how you want your life to be. It takes up disk space, it requires regular maintenance. How great would it be if you could delete all that stuff (properly limited by the commands in this track)? How would you experience the sensation of having a clear mind, positive thoughts and unlimited energy to devote to your weight loss goal? Or, to put it another way, what have you got to lose?

In my work with helping people lose weight, this question poses an interesting dilemma. Should you change the contents of your mind? Is it ethical and appropriate to make these fundamental adjustments to the quality and quantity of your thoughts? Even if the intention is positive?

Think on this. Every moment of everyday you are *already* changing the contents of your mind simply by being awake and taking in all the information that you are bombarded with from all sources as you go about your daily life. Everything you experience during your day is recorded and stored and used to amend your inner world. It already happens automatically. And unfortunately, the changes are usually negative.

Purposefully clearing out the negative from your mind is a positive thing. A lovely thing. You will enjoy it. However, know and understand you will always have control over the process. In order to run this program you will have to say or think the command phrase.

The next stage of the guided meditation in this track includes more limits and safety features. It is spoken in the first person, directly to yourself. "I will limit the operation of this program to 50,000 recorded memories each and every time I run this program while I sleep." And: "I will retain and support all thoughts, memories emotions, beliefs, behaviors and subconscious programs which are necessary for my survival and security in this life." This process is under your control, limited by the command phrase and the numerical limits embedded in the track. The final part of this section is an instruction to trace any of these issues back to a root cause or contributing factor. This includes any past life or cellular memory. Your mind will know if there are any lingering past life or cellular memories that require a clean-up.

REAFFIRM YOUR COMMITMENT TO YOUR GOALS

When the program runs following your command, "SLIM WHILE YOU SLEEP," which you say or think before you go to sleep, your mind will follow the instructions, searching through your recorded memories and neutralizing the negative thoughts, mental blocks, unhelpful beliefs and obstructive behaviors, as you have instructed.

> "Subconscious mind, with this program now successfully in-stalled, you will now RUN this program on my command — SLIM WHILE YOU SLEEP. Subconscious mind, you keep me safe and protected, always doing the best for me. I will repay your faith in me by giving 100% towards achieving our goal of a slim, healthy body for life. I re-affirm my instruction to run this program automatically, every time I sleep when I command you to do so."
>
> — *Slim While You Sleep*, Track 6

When all the instructions have been given and you have successfully designed, installed and run the program, you are then invited to get ready to sink down into sleep. "Very soon you will arrive at the misty borders of sleep. Sleep is your time of relaxation, restoration and re-sourcefulness. Adjust your sleeping position. Get ready to go deeper." There follows about 15 minutes of deeply restful sounds which are designed to lead you into sleep. You can choose to remove your headphones at any time during this phase of the track and drift off to sleep when you are ready.

HOW TO USE THIS TRACK IN PRACTICE

I have designed this track so that once you have installed the program, it runs whenever you sleep *but only when you say the command phrase at bedtime*. I suggest, for the sake of thoroughness, that you should listen to the track *five times* for the installation to be completed. While some people may be very receptive to the suggestions and feel ready to use the command phrase at once, I prefer to err on the side of caution and suggest you listen five times over a short period of time.

Once you have installed the program you can simply go to sleep normally. You now have a sleeping-time subconscious program to run. Your mind already has many interesting sorting programs to run as part of its normal activities, including giving you amazing dreams to inspire you. This program will not add a great deal to the workload. You command your mind to run this sleeping-time program by saying or thinking the words, "SLIM WHILE YOU SLEEP." It is important to have control, to have limits. Therefore, you will be in charge of when you wish to run this program. If it were me, I'd run the subconscious program every night for two weeks and then review how that feels. It only takes a moment to whisper, say, or think the four command words at bedtime. All the hard work has been done for you.

When you wake up and go about your daily life, I'd expect you to feel exactly the same as you usually do. Your sleep should be deeper and more refreshing. You may not notice much difference in the quality of your thoughts. Until, that is, you are in a situation where you would normally expect your mind to try and defeat you. This might be a time when you would typically give in to temptation or eat something you don't want or need. You wait for the negative thinking, the self-talk that is intended to undermine you or make you feel bad about yourself. You may not notice any difference at first, but soon you'll become aware of the peacefulness of your mind, the absence of the usual negative chatter, and the space where there used to be self-limiting beliefs and obstructive behaviors. It may feel like a penny is dropping, or a light is shining. It's hard to define the feeling of knowing that something you used to take for granted isn't there anymore. If you are standing in front of the bakery window, looking at the fattening cakes, waiting for your mind to tell you to go ahead and eat all you want — and you wait — you're expecting the signal to go ahead and ruin your diet, but nothing happens. Your mind is peaceful and full of positive thinking, That's when you'll smile to yourself and understand the benefits of using this track.

I recall, many years ago, working with an elderly lady who had lost her husband and had struggled to recover. They had planned a wonderful retirement but he was taken from her too suddenly and too soon. This lady learned and used a similar technique which neutralizes negative thoughts and emotions. She was working on bringing more joy into her life and letting go of the sadness and grief. At the end of one of her sessions, she stood up and began looking around the room. She then patted her jacket pockets and looked puzzled. She said, "I feel as if I've lost something." We checked the sofa and she looked in her handbag. Then she looked straight into my eyes and said, "I know what it is, I've lost my sadness." And in that moment she understood the purpose of all the therapy and homework she had been doing. I felt a lump in my throat. That is the power of this technique. You can change everything about the way you think about food, your weight loss program and your sense of self. All you have to do is use this track wisely and think or say the command phrase at bedtime.

When you are using this subconscious program, you will soon realize you are thinking differently and acting differently. How you think, of course, will be unique to you. But inside, a powerful positive force has been awakened. You have taken control of the *quality* of your thoughts.

I hope you enjoy this *Slim While You Sleep* track. It is an optional track, so you don't need to use it to have success with your weight loss journey. I have designed it to be powerful, yet simple and quick to use. It would be shame to leave it on the shelf, untried and unused.

CHAPTER 7
OVERCOMING OBSTACLES

"Every now and again, it might feel like you are hitting a wall. There's an obstacle in your way that you don't know how to get around. It can feel frustrating. But with the assistance of your wise inner self, all problems can be transformed into solutions. You can explore those solutions now."

— *Overcoming Obstacles*, Track 7

This verbally-guided meditation is one I use for many therapeutic interventions, and the idea behind it is widely used by many practitioners. It is an inner journey using metaphor, which is designed to be experienced as a lucid dream in a light but focused state of awareness.

The purpose of this meditation is to uncover the meanings behind some of the common obstacles that may frustrate your slimming efforts. You may want to give up, or feel you can't progress any further, or you find yourself sabotaging your efforts. By uncovering the meanings that lie at the heart of these obstacles, you can bring them to conscious awareness, and by doing so you can dissolve their power. Your intelligent mind will also be able to focus on the practical solutions for overcoming whatever the problems represent. When you engage with this process, it can be fascinating to discover what your subconscious mind really thinks about your weight loss plan. It may feel like a light bulb being turned on. "Oh, *that* is what this problem is all about!" A problem you had no idea how to resolve suddenly transforms into a solution. You receive a revelation for you to assimilate and understand. Your "light bulb moment" may have been hiding in plain sight, as if the answer to your problem has been waiting for you to notice it all along.

When you ask your subconscious mind to speak to you, you must be prepared to open your mind and wait for the answer. That is the skill you'll need for this meditation. Insights will be revealed to you which might be in the form of ideas or intuition. You may get an image or a feeling. You will instinctively understand what it all means.

This process is designed to be insightful, but also playful. It should be fun.

SUMMARY OF THE PROCESS
Step 1: Imagining your path and your landscape.
Step 2: Identifying the obstacle in your way.
Step 3: Seeing past it to look at your future.
Step 4: Asking your obstacle to explain itself.
Step 5: Demolishing or removing your obstacle.
Step 6: Walking into your slim, healthy future.

STEP 1: IMAGINING YOUR PATH AND YOUR LANDSCAPE
This track requires you to be awake and aware but relaxed, as though you are in a light daydream. If you slip into a deeper relaxed state you won't be able to follow the instructions. Therefore, this track is best used while in a supported sitting position, and not at bedtime when you are sleepy. Only lie down on a bed if you are confident you won't go too deeply into a meditative state or fall asleep. For that reason, the relaxing introduction is kept short. As long as you can focus inside your mind and stay focused, you'll be fine. The specific Hemi-Sync®

frequencies will enhance and support the correct mind focus for you to enjoy and benefit from this track.

To activate your imagination, you are asked to bring to mind a visual scene — a landscape of your own choosing with a path in it. You are invited to walk along the path. Your mind is perfectly able to do this. If you can dream at night, you can imagine this scene. The important point to remember is not to over-think it. Let images drift into your inner awareness. Remember the sense of playfulness that is fundamental to this guided journey.

Everyone has different ways of imagining things. I have deep respect for those who do not easily visualize, because I am also one of those people. However, it's important to understand that your subconscious mind has a natural ability to work with visual images. Every night you dream in glorious Technicolor®. While you may not always remember your dreams, when you do you'll recall the vivid colorful images you experienced. Therefore, have confidence in your own natural ability to work with visual imagery.

If you struggle with this visualization, then take a few minutes before you begin the track to prepare your mind by imagining visual scenes; remembering scenes from your life, or even by looking at physical images. Think of it as a visual rehearsal.

I once worked with a woman who wanted to experience past life regression. As part of that process, I asked her to open and walk through an imaginary doorway. She explained to me that she was struggling to walk through, the mental images weren't working for her.

We had to find a solution. We stopped and had a short break. I instructed her to practice standing in front of a closed door, then opening it and walking through. She did this several times. This reminded her subconscious mind what we were asking it to do. It gave her something to work with and allowed her to have a successful past life experience.

The imagined path and the landscape in the track are metaphors for what your life is like now. In the same way that you can interpret dreams, similar understanding can be gleaned from the features your imagination chooses to place in this unfolding landscape.

Let your mind fill in all the details. Be open to what you notice. If you stop to do a detailed analysis and interpretation of the scene, you may lose focus. Therefore, tell yourself you can analyze all the different meanings at the end of the track.

Always trust what your inner knowing tells you rather than relying on an external source of dream interpretation.

There are certain accepted dream interpretations that might provide you with some insights, and these are set out below:

THE LANDSCAPE OF YOUR LIFE
- A straight path with grass on either side and no other interesting features — may relate to your life being focused and uncomplicated, but may also indicate life is a bit uninteresting, inflexible, or tightly controlled. You will gain a sense of what it means.
- Meandering path — lots of diversions or complications.
- Hills and valleys — an up-and-down path suggests challenges.
- Trees, flowers and other features — tend to show your life is full of interesting things.
- A desert — depending on how much you like this kind of landscape, this image can suggest a life with little nourishment in it.
- Water — traditionally connected with emotions, depending on what kind of water you see in your landscape. Your mind will give you insight.
- Mountains — can be representative of challenges.

STEP 2: IDENTIFYING THE OBSTACLE IN YOUR WAY

Up ahead there is something in your path, an obstacle or blockage of some kind. The key feature of this blockage is that it's preventing you from moving into your slim, healthy future. Your imagination will supply an image to represent whatever is blocking your progress.

Consider:

- How wide is the blockage? Does it extend to both left and right or does it merely block the path itself?
- How high is it? Can you see over the top?
- What is it made of; what materials?
- Can you see through it?
- Is it immovable, thick and solid, or flimsy and insubstantial?

How you respond to these questions will tell you how significant the blockage is to your progress, and how much work will be required to get through it.

Examples of obstacles:

- A high stone wall, you cannot see over it or around it.
- A brick or block wall, in varying sizes and widths.
- A wooden fence that may be solid or have gaps that you can see through.
- A huge boulder obstructing the path, but not extending far on either side.
- A wall made of hewn timber, like a fort. There may be sharpened spikes on the top.
- A metal gate, like a prison gate.
- An expanse of water.
- A stile.
- A garden gate.
- A ravine.
- Fog or mist.

Allow your mind to choose your own obstacle and decide how wide, tall and impervious it is. You will gain insight from the image about what kind of effort you'll need to put in so you can get past it.

STEP 3: SEEING PAST IT TO LOOK AT YOUR FUTURE

On the other side of this obstacle is your future slim life. Because your imagination is so fantastic, you can float up now and look over the top of your obstacle. You can view the landscape of your future to find out what it is like. You may not need to float. If you can see through your obstacle go ahead and do that. Or go around the side for a peek.

It's important to make sure the imagery is appealing to you. You have the mind power to add in extra features to your future landscape, so go ahead and make it as bright and compelling as you want it to be. You may add more landscape features such as water, trees, flowers and grass. If mountains or valleys appeal to you, you can add these in now. Be bold. The important thing is to understand your power to make your future landscape as wonderful as you want it to be. This is your future in your slim, healthy body. It's where you are headed on this journey. And if you secretly yearn for a shiny red Ferrari, now would be a good time to pop one in your future. You can be as creative as you want to. But remember, the focus of your future is your slim, healthy body. Ferraris can be very distracting.

STEP 4: ASKING YOUR OBSTACLE TO EXPLAIN ITSELF

"As this is an imaginary exercise, this wall or obstacle can speak directly to you, and tell you what it means. Empty your mind and ask this question — what do you represent in my life? Your wise inner self with assist with this process."

— *Overcoming Obstacles*, Track 7

Be patient at this point in the track. Be prepared for some intuition or a fleeting idea. You may get some words right away. There is no right or wrong way to do this. As you practice you will get better every time at listening to what your subconscious mind wants to tell you. Even if you receive no verbal response, the metaphor of the imagery you have conjured up will help you to gain more insight. Your impression of how challenging it will be to get past this obstacle will also help to find out what it represents.

Give yourself a minute or so and keep your conscious mind out of it, because it may want to jump in and supply something logical to fill the silence. The music will aid your listening by getting your mind into the best state to receive any insights or understandings.

STEP 5: DEMOLISHING OR REMOVING YOUR OBSTACLE
This is where the fun begins. You can now choose your destruction method, or call on any demolition equipment that takes your fancy. Get creative. Be as bold as you like. The full range of heavy demolition equipment is available to you. No hire charges. You can imagine you have the services of a deconstruction operator, if you wish. Alternatively, you can try working that wrecking ball yourself. Explosives are good, too. Choose whatever *you* need.

This part of the process can also provide some interesting insights. The ease with which you can remove this obstacle tells you something about how much of a challenge it really will be in your everyday life. Your obstacle may look huge from where you are standing now, but how much effort does it actually take (with the right equipment) to get the path ahead totally clear? Allow your mind to give you additional insights into the true size of the challenge. You can then learn how to optimize your ability to overcome whatever is blocking your path.

When you listen again to this track, you can experiment with different equipment to blast your obstacle into oblivion and find out what works best for you. By experimenting in this way you are increasing the resources at your disposal and teaching yourself flexibility in your problem solving. If you are a person who normally tries to overcome problems in your life by using the same methods each time, this experimentation will allow your mind to consider different and more appropriate approaches.

STEP 6: WALKING INTO YOUR SLIM, HEALTHY FUTURE

Now you can walk tall and with confidence into your slim future 12 months ahead. This is a good time period to ensure you will have achieved your dreams. Your subconscious mind and imagination will move you into your future, with the prompting suggestions from the track. This part of the process helps you to complete your vision of what your life will be like when you have achieved your slimming goals.

Do not hold back or limit yourself. Be as creative as you can, but also allow your wise inner self to shine through the scenery, the props, the people and all the features that make up your future life.

Some elements from your imaged future may be symbols of your future slim happiness and you can interpret them as you explore. There is a saying, "Fake it until you make it." The subconscious mind loves to fake it. Imagination, which runs like a river through your mind, has the power to make this future as bright and wonderful and compelling as you want it to be.

The wooden bench I placed in your future is an easy way for you to get to know your new slim body. I included it because I noticed, when I lost a good deal of weight, how bony my rear became. I noticed there was much less padding when I sat down on a wooden park bench. If the bench doesn't work for you, choose another hard seat, and sense and feel your new slim shape.

The prompts used in the track are designed to help your mind make this part of the meditation as resourceful as possible. Focus on the ideas set out below and let your imagination have a free run.

YOUR NEW APPEARANCE

You may already have an image in your mind about how you will look in your slim future. However, now is good time to refine that image. If you have never been slim in your adult life, you may not have a slim memory to work with. Your creative skills will be called upon to supply the visual representation of how you will look. If you struggle to imagine yourself in a slim, healthy body, do some preparation before you listen to the track again. Find an attractive photograph of your face (that you don't mind cutting up) and a suitable magazine.

Choose a body shape you like in the magazine which has the right overall proportions to suit you. Then join the two together on a sheet of paper. Lock the resulting image in your mind. A little realism is good here. It's not a good idea to turn to contemporary fashion magazines for your cut-out images. We know those models are super-skinny. You can have fun doing this, and experiment by trying several different looks. Work out how your slim self will want to look and what style you're aiming for.

If you have the ability, use photo editing software to meld together a head shot and a body shot. Do whatever you want to get the image that your mind likes best. Your smart phone has many apps to help you.

Your mind will then use this image as evidence you are destined for a slim future. It will not be confused by this slim image you have created. With the right suggestions, this image will be lodged deep inside to motivate you, to inspire you and to embed itself into the reality of your future, 12 months from now. Your subconscious mind accepts such things at face value. Make this image real, bright, compelling and believable. Act as if it were already true. There is powerful mind magic at work here. We utilize this magic to get a clear image of your slim future installed in your mind for you to journey towards. Every step will take you closer to that image of yourself.

YOUR HAPPINESS AND SENSE OF ACHIEVEMENT

When you walk into your future scene, the look on your face and the twinkle in your eye will signal that this future is exactly what you wished for. You will understand that you've achieved something really great, and all your hard work and effort has been worth it. You have persisted. You now have iron willpower. All the things you have done to make this new slim self into reality have resulted in this happy, glowing image of yourself. While this album of meditations is designed to make the journey to a slim, healthy body easy and enjoyable for everyone, it still takes time, effort and energy. This slim, healthy future is, therefore, your great achievement and it's worth celebrating in this future scene.

When you get to this stage in the track, you can allow yourself a self-satisfied smile. You have permission to gloat. You can do this privately and keep your feelings to yourself. As your loved ones will be joining you in the next part, you don't necessarily want them to notice you doing this. Family members or friends can sometimes delight in taking you down a peg or two, and we'll deal with how you should approach this issue shortly.

WHAT YOU WEAR

A whole new wardrobe awaits you and, as the sun is shining in this scene, you can wear summer clothes. Notice the details, the shoes or sandals, your hair, the fabric, the colors. The clothing styles you may have avoided in the past are now available to you, and they will look really good. You can also bring out some old favorites from your wardrobe, if you have held on to them and that's what will make you feel good in this scene.

Popping outside of your body to get a good look at yourself is easy when you are in this expanded state of awareness. Enjoy the look of yourself from many angles. Check to see if you look happy. Make that smile on your face even wider. You deserve it.

JOIN THE PARTY

Bring in all the important people in your life. They want to see you and speak with you. This is your big reveal. Family members and loved ones know how much this means to you and have been with you on your journey. They know what it has taken for you to achieve your slim, healthy body.

Friends or family members or colleagues might want to take you to one side and ask for your secrets. You can explain to them how you have lost your unwanted weight and how much effort you have put in. You can explain what it feels like to have iron willpower. Go ahead and bask in the glory of this feeling. Personalize it. Maybe there is someone who has never believed in you or has sought to undermine you. Bring them in and show them what you have done. Counter any negativity with your wonderful smile and show any doubters you have succeeded. Even if there is a person who has departed this world, you can still call them into this scene.

There is a hypnotherapy treatment called "death bed therapy," where a deceased person is brought to mind for an "honest discussion." When there are unresolved hurts or bad feelings that require resolution, the subconscious mind is a wonderful inner therapy room to make that happen. I was taught to imagine parcel tape over the mouth of the spectral deceased person to stop them from interrupting. No departed souls are harmed by doing this, as it's all done in the imagination. Other forms of gag can be purchased at any hardware store. The client is then encouraged to remove the tape and allow the dead person to have their say. Imagination (or higher connection with spirit) will duly supply some home truths which are invariably wise and healing.

I am writing about this scenario in case it happens spontaneously in your future scene. It might be disconcerting if someone who has brought you down or undermined you turns up in your happy future, either dead or alive. If this happens, try to use it to your advantage. Remember to keep the conversation in the spirit of empowerment, which is what this track is all about.

You can invite anyone you want. Go ahead and call in everyone you wish to show off to. Keep focused on that sense of pride about what you have achieved. Be generous in your praise for those who have supported you.

As you make this scene rich with detail you are, again, setting this future into your mind as if it is already your destiny. Your subconscious mind has a fairly loose grasp of time. By making this future real, compelling and full of wonderful detail, your mind will install it like a memory.

SET THE SCENE INTO YOUR MIND

"When you are happy you have explored everything you want to, imprint this memory as a beautiful movie, with sound and feelings included. Now store it inside your mind where you can revisit it whenever you wish. You have *enacted* a slim, healthy future for yourself, and you will now *walk right into it*. Every step you take from now on will guide you, automatically, towards this wonderful slim future."

— Overcoming Obstacles, Track 7

When you listen to this track regularly you may find different things occur to you along the way. It is an interactive experience. You will receive insights, wisdom and problem resolution as part of the process. Each obstacle you encounter may tell you a different story. You will become so good at demolition that you may consider a career change!

Once you have set this slim, healthy future scene in your mind, your entire self, body, mind and spirit will then walk right towards it, without deviating. You will do this automatically because your mind believes 100% that your slim future is already written.

Motivation is one of the skills of willpower. It can be defined as: "The energy of your incentives to be slim and healthy, to love yourself and your life. You can *see yourself in your slim future and it inspires you.*"

This obstacle-removing track builds up your motivation. By having a clear image of what your future holds, your motivational energy will grow, making you even more unstoppable.

FOLLOWING UP ON THE INSIGHTS FROM THE TRACK
This track is your chance to speak directly to your subconscious mind and to listen to what it has to say. The details of the conversation will be in the form of the images, metaphors and symbols you receive as well as a few well-chosen words about what your obstacle represents in your life.

I'm confident you will gain insights to go with the images as you go along. Don't over-think it. It is not a logical process. By bringing subconscious material to the surface, it can be safely resolved, sometimes without any conscious awareness that it's happening.

Large insurmountable obstacles should not be a cause for concern because the imagery may be trying to tell you that the obstacle is large *in your mind*, not in reality. Rely on your inner knowing and approach the process with an open mind.

When you can see through an obstacle, your mind is telling you it's not as significant as you think.

Sometimes the right thing to do is to walk around your obstacle or climb over it. This shows you how easy it can be to get past.

114

When equipment is needed, this can be a sign that extra resources are required to get past this obstacle, either internal or external resources.

An obstacle that extends all the way out of sight to the left and right is likely to be more of a challenge than a blockage that covers only the path.

The effort you put in during the track is a sign of how much effort you need to get past this obstacle. However, when you have lined up your demolition method, how easily does the obstacle fall? Does it dissolve quickly? Or do you need to bash out every little part of it? This tells you something about the actual effort you'll have to put in to remove it.

Sometimes you might get a fence but it has barbed wire on it. This tells you getting past will have hidden barbs for you to take care of.

Water obstacles signify emotional challenges in dream interpretation, but be inclined to rely more on the wisdom from your own inner knowing.

If you find your future doesn't look bright or interesting, remember *you* can make this happen deliberately. You are in charge.

As you practice, you'll gain more skill with this form of inner work. As a form of lucid dream that you have control of, you can utilize the various points on the journey to work on other life obstacles that may need resolution.

Making a note of the things you recall will give you reference points to explore during your journey towards a slim, healthy body.

Don't be surprised if you gain more insights while you are going about your daily life. Your mind will work on making sense of everything you have discovered, giving you its verdict at unexpected times.

CHAPTER 8
RELEASE THE PAST

"The past is where you have come from on your life journey, where you have overcome challenges and learned things about yourself. Now is the time to integrate that learning but let go of all the thoughts, beliefs, emotions and memories that are standing in the way of your slim future."

— *Release the Past*, Track 8

Right now, as you are reading this, you are made up of all the memories of everything that ever happened to you. It doesn't matter whether you can remember these life events because your subconscious mind remembers everything. It uses all your experiences to form a clear idea of who you are, how your body works, what you like and dislike, how your emotions function and how you respond to the world around you. Your subconscious mind needs all of this information to help you to get the best out of your life and to *survive*. That is the goal.

And as you read this, you have survived! Considering how tough life can be, you did an excellent job. You relied on the support of your powerful subconscious mind which has all your personal data at its disposal. While you may not feel enthusiastic about where you are in your life, please accept the praise and support that is coming from deep inside. You can give yourself a heartfelt pat on the back for coming this far. You deserve it.

THE PAST CAN AFFECT THE PRESENT

But what if the past and the memories still have the power to affect you in ways that are interfering with your weight loss goals? What if the past is holding you back? Perhaps you are reminded from time to time of past events and you cannot let go of them. You may struggle to consign these memories to the archives in your mind where they no longer have the power to affect you.

This Hemi-Sync® track, *Release the Past* has been designed for you travel back in time, safely and gently, with your wise inner self as a companion. You then work on dissolving the threads that bind you to the past in a safe and constructive manner while still retaining the wisdom from the lessons you learned.

"Your wise self is that part of you that knows you best, your cheerleader, lovingly watching over everything that you do. This self has integrated all the wisdom from everything you have ever experienced, in this life and in all your past, current and future travels in this universe of energy."

— *Release the Past,* Track 8

YOU REMEMBER HOW YOU FELT AT YOUR GOAL WEIGHT

When somebody comes for help with losing weight, one of the questions I ask is, "What is your goal weight, specifically?" The follow-up question is, "How old were you when you were last at that weight and what was happening in your life at the time?"

Take a moment now to think about your exact goal weight. Then go back in time and remember when you were last at that weight. Remember other times when you were at that weight. Then get specific and recall what life events were happening at the time. Was your weight loss a good thing? Were you happy and your weight reflected your state of mind? Or were you in a difficult life situation? Were health concerns connected to your weight loss? Or challenging times in your relationships? Allow yourself a moment to relive some of the emotions from these past times.

I recall a woman who explained, "The last time I was at that weight was when I was getting a divorce. I was totally miserable and couldn't eat." Another client told me, "I last weighed that when I was a teenager. I didn't have a happy time at my school and I try not to think about it."

The past is also where you struggled to lose weight or experienced unpleasant diets or had multiple experiences of failure. Recall how you felt, what you went through, the ups and downs. Remember all the negative things, if it's not too uncomfortable for you. If the mere thought of trying to lose weight makes you feel defeated before you even begin, this feeling most likely comes from your past experiences that carry with them that sense of failure.

When you consider how powerful memories are, it is no wonder that a deep part of you may resist trying to lose weight. Your subconscious mind doesn't want you to be unhappy. It doesn't like it when you are bored with eating dreary diet food, fed up with not enjoying yourself, annoyed you can't go out for meals with friends or when you're sick of feeling hungry.

The past has the power to affect your life choices now. If what happened in the past is stopping you from achieving a slim, healthy body, now is the time to heal all of those memories and begin with a clean slate. While it is important to respect the lessons from the past, you have permission to let go of any emotional threads that are binding you to those past memories. The lessons are for you to make use of *now*, to give you an edge as you move on with your life. The memories are long gone and can be consigned to your archive.

NO MEMORIES OF BEING SLIM

You may not have any clear memories of being slim because you've struggled with your weight for most of your life. With no previous experience to guide you, your imagination must come to the fore. You can easily create an imagined slim past, and this can be a great resource. Start by imagining a believable image of yourself at your perfect weight. Use a photograph of your face and join it to a suitable body cut from a magazine, trying various designs until you get an image you like. Or use your computer with a selection of images to do this electronically. Then design a perfect time in your past, an interlude where you were living your best slim life. This will enable your mind to have something firm to focus on when you are considering what your life will be like. This imagined picture of your slim self will also come in handy to inspire you for the *Overcoming Obstacles* track, when you are asked to travel into your slim future and imagine what life will be like. Simply by flexing and exercising your imagination you are doing something positive, and setting your intention to achieve that slim, healthy body you wish for.

PAST EVENTS THAT CAUSED WEIGHT GAIN

It's likely that events in the past made you gain weight. Such events are not always connected with emotional eating. I recall a slim woman who had a car accident and had to spend many months in recovery. To her intense annoyance, she gained 30 pounds. There was nothing she could do about it. By the time she had recovered, she was overweight and felt bad about her body. It would take many more months of effort to slim down and regain her health.

Another example is a man who had to travel abroad for part of the year, away from his family while working on a business project. He stayed in hotels and ate too much food. There were compulsory business and social engagements to attend. He had few opportunities to stay active and eat healthily. He felt stressed and lonely. Weight gain followed.

Women typically gain weight when they have babies. Nature has its own agenda and hormones play a part. Men tend to gain weight when they are looked after by loving wives or partners. Happiness can make you forget to watch your food intake. By the time you look at yourself in the mirror, you have gained a lot of weight. Therefore, past life events that do not necessarily have a negative emotional element can be the source of weight gain. And happiness invariably makes you forget about your waistline.

However, one thing is certain. It will take effort and energy to lose that weight because experience tells us it's unlikely to dissolve by itself.

PAST EMOTIONS CAN BE TO BLAME

The past is also where you experienced emotional upheaval and this may have led to weight gain. In the past, there may have been relationships that didn't work out and the strain made you eat more. Those extra pounds are still there, reminding you of those times. In the past you perhaps struggled with jobs you didn't like, and those feelings made you eat to get through the day. When you finally found a career that fulfilled you, the extra weight stayed put.

In the past, you may have faced all that life can throw at you, enduring grief and hurt, sadness and loneliness, doubts and fears, stress and pressure and life events that spiraled out of control. Sometimes the only way to get through and safely out to the other side is to eat. But when the extra weight lingers after your life has been fixed, it can seem very unfair. Excess weight tends to have stubborn, glue-like qualities.

At this moment in your life you could be happy and fulfilled having learned all you need from life's challenges, yet the pounds you put on as a response to those struggles still linger on, grumpy and wobbling, waiting to be shed. Your current satisfaction with your life isn't shining out, bright and beautiful. You cannot show the world how great you feel about your life if you still have that excess weight hanging around.

HUMAN DNA IS PROGRAMMED FOR SURVIVAL

While we are considering the effect of the past on your body weight now, it's also worth considering the influence of humankind's history on this planet. Our ancestors survived because they developed creative ways to feed themselves across many different terrains and climates. Starvation was an everyday reality. Populations moved to different continents in search of food supplies. It's easy to forget the influence of the past and food scarcity when you have a supermarket around the corner from your house.

The past, with all its survival challenges, is integrated into our DNA code at a deep level. Human beings have been programmed over thousands of years to be miserly with energy usage. If your genetic inheritance includes a body design that stored fat in times of plenty, you would have survived to become the next generation. Skinny humans whose bodies frittered energy away would not have been able to survive tough times. I sometimes console myself with this thought.

PAST LIVES OF STRUGGLE

A further aspect of the past that may influence your weight now is your memories of former incarnations. Past life memories, in other words. While some may think the concept of past lives is unscientific or unbelievable, it is worth exploring in case it does apply to you. If you have lived in other bodies in the past, it's statistically likely you experienced lives where struggling to eat enough was an important feature. The vast majority of our ancestors knew about starvation, disease and death. If you endured such lives in the past, there is some logic to the idea that a deep part of you may resist attempts to lose weight on purpose. You may not know where this feeling of reluctance comes from. It may feel subtle, imperceptible, hard to pin down, like an emotional cloud that surrounds you. Past life memories can transmit energetic messages that influence behavior in your current life and act as blocks to success. Past life or current life memories can all be considered together using the broad definition of "the past." Healing all of it collectively will ensure there are no barriers standing in your way to frustrate all your weight loss efforts.

The following example of the influence of past life memories sticks in my mind. I knew a woman who, for no logical reason, felt compelled to keep kitchen cupboards stocked to bursting with food, much more food than her family could eat. This behavior came into sharp focus during times when her family enjoyed self-catering vacations. The first thing on the to-do list was to visit the supermarket and stock the empty cupboards up. She always bought much more than was required for the duration of the holiday. It became a family joke. If there was no supermarket or food store in easy reach, serious anxiety would kick in. The behavior only manifested itself after the children were born. Her husband reminded her about the empty refrigerator when he first met her. "One yogurt, some milk and a tin of cat food, that's all the food you kept in the house. Not enough to keep a fly alive," he had joked.

Past life regression revealed a life as a widow with young children, hungry and struggling to survive. The children died first. She recalled her last day on earth, starving and grief-stricken. She gave up her life, having no will to continue. The emotional trauma from recalling that life stayed with her for many days. It took several weeks to assimilate the understandings from those terrible memories. The therapeutic result was that the compulsion to overfill cupboards dissolved naturally as part of the process. This had not been her aim when the regression was planned. She only reported it as an interesting side effect of releasing the past life energy. The worry about not getting enough to eat also dissolved. She could relax into a weight loss plan.

Her fear of not having enough food to stave off starvation had safely resolved itself.

The treatments for problems caused by past life memories and genetic survival instincts are identical to the treatment for any problems caused by current life memories. Simply by bringing the emotions or thoughts or impressions up to conscious awareness, they can dissipate. Thinking about them, understanding them and analyzing them *dissolves their power*. When you pay attention to these messages from deep inside, your subconscious mind can heave a sigh of relief, knowing you are fully on board with all its worries. It can stand down from its state of high alert. You will have reassured your subconscious mind that you can be trusted not take unnecessary risks with your life and put your survival in jeopardy. Your logical conscious mind then jumps for joy. By journeying towards a slim, healthy body you are putting your own health and wellbeing first and ensuring you have the best chance of a long, happy and fulfilling life. No part of your mind could argue with that.

This Hemi-Sync® track will guide you towards uniting your conscious and subconscious minds so that both are working towards the same goal. Simply by listening and acknowledging your subconscious mind's concerns, you can release the energy from the past, memories from all sources, and prevent them from sabotaging your journey towards a slim, healthy future.

YOUR WISE INNER SELF PROTECTS YOU ON THIS JOURNEY
Before you begin, I assure you that you won't be prompted by the verbal guidance to recall specific memories or relive memories that are painful. If your past includes any traumatic events or times of great unhappiness, even if you only suspect you might have these memories inside, have confidence that your wise inner self is always there, ensuring everything goes to plan without unwanted distress. You are always protected in this way when you engage in guided meditation.

> "Now listen carefully. Know that memories are merely made of thought energy charged with emotions. When you work on healing the past, your mind will keep a safe distance from all negative memories. You will receive only a neutral image or a symbol or a fleeting thought, only sufficient to remind you, without any emotional distress, of past events that still have power over you."
>
> — *Release the Past,* Track 8

The image or symbol or fleeting thought that is suggested in the track will be enough to allow healing to take place. For this process to be effective, your wise inner self then travels back in time to provide comfort and reassurance to your younger self. This technique is widely used in therapy and is very useful for all aspects of healing the past.

> "Allow your wise self to travel back in time and comfort you in that memory. To hug you and tell you all will be well. You know this because you are here now in your present, a being shaped and honed and made stronger by everything that has ever happened to you. Sense the comfort, notice the healing and any binding threads dissolve into mist."
>
> — *Release the Past,* Track 8

You will be prompted to think about events from the past, but in a safe way. You will be encased in a cocoon of light energy that you have invited to form a protective shield around you. From the safety of your cocoon, and by viewing the past from a distance, no negative energy can affect you. It is as if you are a dispassionate bystander, observing, learning and neutralizing past hurts. You are reminded that memories are merely made of thought energy charged with emotions. While such memories were overwhelming at the time, by observing from a safe distance you are disconnected from any emotional distress. As you work on this healing, the symbolic threads that bind you to your past are dissolved. You then send the neutralized memories to a place of absolute safety in your mind. During the track you are prompted to do this three times. That will be sufficient work for each time you listen.

REWRITE THE EMOTION OF YOUR MEMORIES

Your wise inner self, by taking on the role of comforter and supporter for your younger self, also provides the energy to heal the hurt in retrospect. It will seem as if you really had that comfort at the time of the past event. It will be as if the memory has been re-written with a more positive outcome. This Hemi-Sync® track, by working on so many levels, has the power to heal, comfort and re-imagine your past so it loses all power to affect you now.

You may want to listen to the track several times to derive the full benefits. Because this verbally-guided meditation is an interactive track, you will gain best results by remaining aware as you listen. This is not a track for falling asleep, as you won't have awareness of the stages as you progress. There are other tracks for bedtime, such as the *Slim While You Sleep* track.

"You are made stronger, more experienced, more resourceful from the memories of everything that has ever happened to you."

— *Release the Past,* Track 8

THE POWER OF INTENTION

There are other benefits from actively healing the past. When you decide to move forward in your life (as opposed to dwelling on past hurts) you are giving your mind an important message. You are saying "thank you" for its useful contribution, but now you are going to take back control. Your *intention* is to move forward and leave the past with all its hurts, traumas and distress, behind you. This signals to your mind that you mean business. In the field of complementary therapy this phenomenon is called *intentionality.* It represents a huge energy change inside you.

When you intend to change you move all of your stuck energy out of the way, allowing more positive thinking and momentum to take its place. Whenever you put on one of the Hemi-Sync® tracks, you are signaling to your subconscious mind that you are no longer prepared to go on like this. You want to change, and you command your mind to accept that you want to change.

This track can be used as often as you wish. Think of the benefits — by neutralizing the past you begin to wipe the slate clean and start afresh. You will have more energy to devote to your goals because you won't have to waste any energy on the past.

CHAPTER 9
SELF-SABOTAGE

"The human mind and emotional system is complex. Any journey towards a desired goal may be characterized by doubts and fears along the way. Sometimes those powerful emotions trigger a response called self-sabotage. It may seem as if you have two distinct selves, arguing with each other and pulling in different directions."

— *Self-Sabotage,* Track 9

Self-sabotage sounds dramatic and serious, but it's not. It is a familiar and completely normal human response and you may notice it in everyday life, in your own behavior and in the behavior of others. It's important to find out more about this phenomenon because, for those who want to get slim and healthy, self-sabotage is a deal-breaker. It's a problem that needs to be fixed. The introduction to this Hemi-Sync® track talks about two distinct selves arguing with each other. One part wants to follow a particular path and the other part is determined to do the opposite, pulling you in different directions. That is what it can feel like — being pulled apart in an internal psychological fight.

This phenomenon can be puzzling because the source of the conflict is so illogical. You *know* you want to achieve a slim, healthy body but you still keep on sabotaging your best efforts. Think about some simple examples that illustrate self-sabotage:

- Buying your favourite diet-busting food when you know very well you will eat it the moment you get the chance.
- Going out for drinks then being persuaded to go for a meal afterwards even though your hunger will make you overeat.
- Your fridge is empty so you use this as an excuse to order a takeout meal.
- Attending a family function with an empty stomach and then hitting the buffet with a vengeance.

These examples show how you can fool yourself into believing you have no choice, yet with a little planning, the sabotaging of your weight loss plans could be prevented.

SELF-SABOTAGE — CONFLICT ABOUT WHAT'S BEST FOR YOU

A more frustrating example of diet self-sabotage happens when you are losing weight well, feeling great and you are happy with your progress. You are on track and you feel in control. Success may be within reach. Then, without warning, something snaps. All that good work is lost. You go right back to your old ways of overeating and put all the weight back on. It's inexplicable and you may not understand what is happening. This type of self-sabotage is likely to be rooted in a psychological battle between your conscious mind and your subconscious mind.

The conflict arises because you have decided to make far reaching life changes. You have decided this *consciously*. The conscious part of your mind has used logic and reason to make the decision to lose weight. You know it's the best thing for you. You know you will benefit. All the evidence suggests it. You will feel better and are likely to enjoy greater wellbeing if you are slim and healthy. So far, so good. You then choose a plan, make changes to your diet, decide what you'll eat and how much activity you'll do. You keep track of your progress on the scales. You measure your body and jot down how many inches you've lost. You may take photos of your changing shape. These are all conscious functions. You continue to lose weight and you are happy with your progress. There is no logical reason for you to give up.

Deep inside, your subconscious mind is quietly monitoring these developments. It's going along with the weight loss plan, grudgingly, but it has suspicions that this life change may not be good for you. As far as your subconscious mind is concerned, eating less and losing weight may raise a warning flag. There might be safety and security issues involved. What if this part of your mind had secret information that it believed conflicted with your weight loss plan? Or what if it believed that overeating was the best way to keep you safe from all kinds of harm in this difficult life? It sounds illogical, but judgment and logic are not your subconscious mind's strong points.

When your subconscious mind decides it's time to take action to stop you getting slim and healthy, it can exert a powerful influence on your behavior. You may experience a gnawing sense that something is wrong, but you can't put your finger on what might be. You may not notice anything different except that you no longer feel enthusiastic about losing weight and your willpower flies out of the window. Why would your subconscious mind frustrate your efforts in this underhand way?

LIFE CAN BE HARD AND A GOOD COPING STRATEGY IS NEEDED
There is an irony in this mental conflict. All your subconscious mind is trying to do is to keep you safe from all of life's hurts and challenges and pitfalls. From an early age, its job has been to help you find ways of coping with everything that life can throw at you. Even if your upbringing was totally comfortable, stable and happy, there will have been hurts and disappointments you had to deal with. Human life is

like that. For the majority of us, our early lives had many difficult patches. Simply going through the teens is a huge life challenge in itself. Therefore, a really good *coping strategy* needs to be worked out. Your subconscious mind will choose a coping strategy that works to help with life's ups and downs, smoothing over the bad times until better times come along. And there are so many different ways to choose from to cope with life's challenges. Some ways work better than others. Some ways of coping with the tough times can ultimately be self-destructive. Addictions to drugs, alcohol and gambling fall into this category. For a coping strategy to work, it has be easy to use and appropriate to the circumstances, without too many negative side-effects.

As an effective coping strategy, eating delicious food has got to be right up there near the top of the list. It activates all of your pleasure sensors and you get a wonderful release of "feel good" chemicals inside you. Not only that, eating acts as a powerful distraction from whatever is bothering you. Delicious food is freely available to buy, totally legal and reasonably inexpensive. Eating is also socially acceptable, a normal part of everyday life. Eating is so absorbing, it's hard to feel anxious or worried or hurt or distressed while you are doing it. Therefore, it's perfectly possible that eating is a great choice as a coping strategy for the majority of problems that human beings will encounter. If eating is your way of coping with life, your subconscious mind soon locks that idea into its toolbox as its #1 way of keeping you safe and protected from unnecessary hurts.

It's no accident that people gain weight when they are under stress. Tough times call for tough measures and you may automatically reach for comforting food when you need something extra to help you cope. Your subconscious mind, in its role as your protector, would prefer that you gain weight and cope with your problems, rather than teeter on the brink of that deep, dark hole that it worries about. A little extra weight doesn't bother it at all. It's a minor irrelevance. The coping habits of childhood and your teens years soon become ingrained. Eating becomes your preferred way of coping and it will get you through to better times, even if you are not aware that you are using food as an emotional anesthetic or a distraction technique.

Think about how your weight has fluctuated in good times and bad. There may be a direct correlation between weight gain and the tough times in your life. The converse can also be true. Many people report they also overeat when times are good, when wonderful life events happen. A common example is when you settle down into life with a beloved partner. There is a good reason why extra weight around the waist is called "love handles." It's almost as if your subconscious says to you: "Hooray! You can relax now because you're in love and therefore you are safe and happy and protected, which is what I wanted for you all along."

YOUR MIND THEN RAISES A RED FLAG

Some way along your journey towards a slim, healthy body, you may reach a point where your subconscious mind gets seriously annoyed. You are willfully ignoring its #1 belief that overeating is necessary to keep you safe and protected. You are messing with the basic survival strategy that it has devised for you. No wonder the red flag is raised. This acts as a call to action. And without quite understanding why this is happening, you subconsciously begin to sabotage yourself.

There are many variations of self-sabotaging behavior that people exhibit in their lives. It's a natural part of being human. Sometimes it turns out that the sabotage is essential to stop you from doing something crazy. It can work like this: occasionally your logical conscious self hatches ambitious life changes that will put you at serious risk of failure and harm. "Why don't you give up work and become a professional sky-diver," it says. Or, "Why don't you mortgage yourself up to the hilt and buy that beautiful house you want?" At such times, the protective subconscious will do its sabotaging work beautifully and keep you awake at night, tossing and turning, sleepless with worry, until you give up your impetuous plans.

Navigating through life's challenges requires the two parts of your mind to co-operate and work together in a harmonious way, rather that fighting with each other. The aim of this track is to heal the differences of opinion and bring understanding and harmony in its place. The verbal guidance will speak directly to your subconscious mind, giving it reassurance that what you wish for is good for you, beneficial to your wellbeing and that losing weight will ensure you are safe and protected. Losing weight may actually help you cope better with life's tough times. Your confidence will improve, you'll feel good about yourself and you'll feel more in control of your life. You'll be empowered and full of energy. It's impossible to overestimate what a positive difference this journey towards a slim, healthy body will make to you. That's a message your subconscious mind must fully under-stand and agree to abide by.

UNITING IN A SPIRIT OF CO-OPERATION

When you listen to this gentle, but healing, guided meditation, you're invited to use visualization to teach your subconscious mind about your new plans for your slim, healthy life. If a picture paints a thousand words, then using this visualization will send an unequivocal message to your misinformed subconscious mind and challenge it to get onto the exact same page as your logical conscious mind.

The imagery encourages you to visualize yourself internally as two distinct selves. One is made of bright yellow light, full of positivity and energy. The other self is grey, weighed down with negative thinking and always worrying about the worst that can happen. You talk directly to your grey self and reassure it that all will be well. You tell it honestly that you know what you are doing. Getting slim and healthy will be right for you. You therefore bring the potential conflict between your two inner selves up into conscious awareness.

> "One of your selves, the energetic, proactive self is made of glowing yellow light. It is ready to get on with the business of improving your life. The other self is made of grey light, lacking in positivity, always seeing the pitfalls and problems."
>
> — *Self-Sabotage*, Track 9

Using this track is no different to having an honest heart-to-heart with a loved one. In this case, that loved one is your deep subconscious. It needs to understand from the source (you) that you take full responsibility for the decision to stop overeating to compensate for all of life's problems.

> "Open my heart to the possibilities of living a slim, healthy life. I know there may be challenges, ups and downs. I am ready. I am not scared. I will live a slim, healthy life. It is my goal. It requires everything I have to give. Fear of failure will not stop me from achieving this in my life."
>
> — *Self-Sabotage*, Track 9

When your grey self merges with your yellow self and is transformed, the healing messages will spread throughout all parts of your mind including your emotions, your memories, your behaviors and your beliefs about yourself. This simple imagery can therefore be a visual talisman for you as you carry on your journey towards a slim, healthy body. You can fix the image in your mind and revisit it from time to time to remind you about your commitment to go forward in positive yellow light.

Once you have grasped this idea of how self-sabotage works and you have brought the actuality of it into conscious awareness, you are armed and ready to ensure you never again fall into the trap of pressing the "stop" button on your dreams for your future life whether it is by accident or design. It will be an ongoing process. It may take time to build the right level of internal trust. All the guided meditations in this album will support you along the way.

ARE YOU WORRIED WHAT IT WILL FEEL LIKE TO SUCCEED?

In Track 7, *Overcoming Obstacles*, you are invited to travel forwards in time into an imaginary future to explore the experience of having a slim, healthy body. By building layer upon layer of future "memories" about how amazing your life will be when you've achieved your goals, you are imprinting a slim future into your mind *as if it was already your destiny*.

You can practice making your future brighter, more realistic and more appealing every time you use the track. You can play with it and have lots of fun. You're telling your mind that your slim future will be something to really look forward to.

Sometimes the idea of success gives rise to mixed feelings. Success has an exact opposite — failure. If you have struggled with your weight in the past, it's likely that you've experienced what it feels like to fail. It's disheartening when this happens once or twice but it's not the end of the world. You dust yourself off and try again. However, if you keep on failing, no matter how hard you try, you'll wear down your store of that important positive energy you need to keep on trying. Nobody likes to fail. Giving up is not something that is highly valued in our modern society. Everywhere you turn in all forms of media you will encounter unrelenting messages about "never giving up" or "keep on pushing" or "come back fighting." After a while such phrases cease to be motivating when your mind can't relate those messages to your own experiences.

It follows that self-sabotage can also be a result of what we might call *failure fatigue*. It's really hard to keep getting back up and trying again over and over if the end result is still failure. You need to keep your self-respect intact so the only course open to you is to step away and simply stop trying. At this point your mind is activating its natural self-protection strategy. By not giving 100%, by not really trying, you can always convince yourself you failed because you didn't try hard enough. You can reassure yourself that you *could* have succeeded if you *had* tried. What you need to combat failure fatigue and go on to succeed is extra resources. The 12 emotionally nourishing tracks in this album will provide all the resources you require.

Nevertheless, you must be *prepared to try*. Giving 100% to this process will ensure success, even if you have failed over and over in the past. I have unshakeable faith that you will succeed because this 12 track album is a feast of weight loss support with an abundance of powerful resources that will reverse whatever has been stopping you from losing weight and creating that slim, healthy body you deserve. Yes, I really do mean you deserve it. Even if you have a multitude of doubts or are convinced you will fail.

"You will never be frightened of failing and allow that fear to stop you trying. If you stumble, you'll get right up and carry on. You'll put 100% effort into all that you do."

— *Self-Sabotage*, Track 9

In order to achieve success, all you have to do is to try. Listen to the tracks, as often as is described in the instructions. Learn more about this inner work you are doing by studying this book. Absorb new understandings about yourself. Commit to putting 100% effort in, no excuses. If those ideas send a shiver of fear through you (for all the reasons I've described) know that there is a simple and healing antidote which is included in this track and is the foundation of the affirmations used in this album.

The antidote to failure fatigue is simple — you begin to give yourself positive messages of praise. You learn how to praise yourself in words that make you feel good. Then you practice giving yourself praise and compliments, over and over, until it becomes your habit. The positive dialogue with yourself will easily counteract any doubts and fears about trying, and failing. Giving yourself praise and compliments may be new to you. It may feel strange at first. Practice makes perfect, however, and you'll soon get the hang of it. The affirmations of praise in the verbal guidance include a pause between each phrase so you can repeat it, in your head or out loud.

I challenge you to lavish compliments on yourself. Counteract the negative thinking, the doubts, the internal criticism. Soon it will feel normal to receive these compliments and the words will permeate into your normal everyday internal chatter. Which is exactly how it should be.

"You will now make a vow to yourself to communicate all your inner thoughts with a positive voice at all times. From now on, you will send yourself messages of support every day. Messages of appreciation. And little by little, you will make this into your new habit."

— *Self-Sabotage,* Track 9

You are hereby charged with the task of being your own inner cheer-leader. We already know this is the main job of your wise inner self. If you've been ignoring the inner cheering from this part of you, now it's time to get on the same side and shout your praise and compliments louder. You need to hear them. You may also have to work on *accepting* this praise. Stop for a moment and think about how you react if somebody praises you or gives you a compliment. Do you evade the praise? Or disagree with it? Or do you bask in it and accept it with a proud, "Thank you."

Make a decision now to thank your wise inner self when it gives you the compliments from this track and when it showers you with spontaneous praise in the future. A heart-felt "thank you" will then act as a sign that you are united in your common purpose, healed with bright yellow light and completely infused with the energy of success. This is also the energy of giving 100% of your effort.

This self-sabotage track tackles a difficult subject. It may sting a little when you think about it. However, the guided meditation is filled with all things healing and positive to help you make self-sabotage a thing of the past.

Listen to this track as often as you need to. Reaffirm your commitment to giving this process 100% of your effort and energy. You will be rewarded by benefits that spread out into other parts of your life.

Once you've learned all you need from this track, the *Affirmations for a Slim, Healthy Body* in Track 11 will continue to give you plenty of practice in talking to yourself in positive, supportive ways.

To finish on this subject, you can adapt the acutapping procedure in Track 4, *Craving Control*, to help you let go of self-sabotaging thoughts and emotions. The phrases have been adapted to focus on reversing self-sabotage. Before you practice this acutapping procedure, refresh your memory of the points by looking again at Chapter 4 or the instructions in the brochure. You can say the generic phrase, such as the one written out in the example that follows. When you have more confidence in your understanding of yourself, you can design your own accompanying phrases to fulfill your own needs. The tapping points and sequence remain the same.

When you practice acutapping regularly, you are stimulating your inner life force energy while thinking or speaking the phrases that resonate with you. In the procedure that follows, you are instructed to *release the negative* which is how acutapping phrases are normally designed. You then state a positive phrase. This mixture of negative and positive has the effect of making your mind choose between negative thoughts about yourself and the opposite, which is to embrace the wonderful statement: "I am worthy of compliments." Given such a choice, your mind will make the right one. This positive statement will travel like an arrow, deep into your belief system.

FULL ANTI-SABOTAGE ACUTAPPING PROCEDURE:

Get comfortable, sitting down with your legs uncrossed in a reasonably upright position.

1. Begin tapping your *eyebrow point*, and repeat these words as you tap: "I release all the negative ways I talk to myself inside. I am worthy of compliments."

2. Now to the *side eye point*, tap it and say: "I release all the negative ways I talk to myself inside. I am worthy of compliments."

3. Now to the *under eye point*, tap and say: "I release all the negative ways I talk to myself inside. I am worthy of compliments."

4. Now to the *under nose point*, tap and say these words: "I release all the negative ways I talk to myself inside. I am worthy of compliments."

5. Now to the *collarbone point*, tap with 3 fingers, while you say: "I release all the negative ways I talk to myself inside. I am worthy of compliments."

6. Now to the *index finger point*. You say: "I release all the negative ways I talk to myself inside. I am worthy of compliments."

7. Now to the *little finger point*. Tap and say: "I release all the negative ways I talk to myself inside. I am worthy of compliments."

8. Finally, take hold of your hand, and press the *center of your palm* with your thumb, and say: "I release all the negative ways I talk to myself inside. I am worthy of compliments."

Breathe in and out. You are sending a strong message to your inner self to free yourself from whatever is holding you back. Take a deep breath, wait a few moments, then start again. Practice this acutapping sequence and gain maximum effectiveness by working on one phrase at a time, for about five minutes, before moving on to the next phrase. A good acutapping session will last about 15 minutes. You should feel a sense of release, of lightness. The more you work at this, the better you will feel.

If you want to be more precise about your own self-sabotaging thoughts or behaviors, you can design a suitable phrase and make it *specific to you*, incorporate the *positive* and express it in the *first person*. First, concentrate on what you want to let go of. Use the words you would normally use to express your thoughts and feelings. You end each phrase with a short positive sentence. For example:

- I release the fear that I'll fail at this weight loss journey. I am full of courage.
- I let go of the worry that I'll sabotage myself. I'm confident I'll succeed.
- I am free from the feeling of wanting to give up. I commit to keep going.
- I release the thought that I'm scared of giving 100%. I am unafraid.
- I let go of my habit of pressing the "self-destruct" button when things are going well. I love to persevere.
- I am free from the fear of failing at anything I do. I am brave and fearless.

When you have worked at one or two of your phrases for about 15 minutes (or however much time you have available), take a moment to notice the energy buzzing inside you. Aside from working to reverse self-sabotage, this simple technique can be used to get your energy moving and sparkling anytime, anywhere. When you have learned the acutapping procedure and no longer have to refer to the notes, you can multi-task by doing it whenever you get the chance. You can repeat the words silently if this is better for you. Try and find time to practice when you have some spare minutes during your day.

- When you are waiting for the kettle to boil.
- While the shower warms up.
- During ad-breaks on the TV.
- When you get out of bed.
- When you have finished getting dressed.
- Before or after meals.
- When you need a boost mid-afternoon.
- When you get home from work.

Surprise yourself with how energized you can feel when you use this technique every day, many times a day.

Dealing with self-sabotage sounds difficult but is surprisingly simple. It involves uniting parts of the mind that have become confused and conflicted and transforming them into healing yellow light. It involves praising yourself in the same way you would praise or compliment a loved one. All the tracks in this album are infused with this special form of language and it's relentlessly positive. You will hear, learn and absorb a multitude of kind words into your normal vocabulary as you progress. Your inner dialogue will soon change and will keep evolving and adapting to whatever wonderful, life-affirming things you choose to do in your future.

A slim, healthy body is your main focus right now, but in the future there will be other ambitious goals for you to aim for. Once you are truly united deep inside, you can be confident that self-sabotage will be a thing of the past.

CHAPTER 10
WALKING MEDITATION

"Walking is a wonderful way to clear your mind, reaffirm your goals, release stress and tension, all while infusing your mind with powerful messages to support your slim, healthy future. Your conscious mind will be engaged in the pleasure of your walk, performing all the necessary physical actions, while your unconscious listens and learns."

— Walking Meditation, Track 10

Walking is something almost everyone can do. It's the simplest form of human exercise. You don't have to think about how to do it or what special equipment is required. Walking comes naturally.

Getting out in the fresh air and experiencing the natural world outdoors brings many health benefits. Even if you live and work in the center of a bustling city, there will be walks you can take that don't expose you to bumper-to-bumper traffic, noise and stress.

Walking is the antidote to an indoor sedentary life. It can undo all the physical problems associated with sitting at a desk and staring at a screen for many hours a day. It can also soothe the mind and body of someone who spends all day on their feet, rushing around. Walking is not the same as standing about or dashing backwards and forwards from place to place, fueled by adrenaline, worrying about deadlines and thinking, thinking, thinking. Walking is also the exact opposite of sitting in a car for long periods of time.

What's more, this simple and beneficial activity, taking no more than 20 minutes of your day, can be used to meditate on all of the positive messages that form the core of this program.

WALKING IS AN ANTIDOTE TO STRESS

I'm reminded of a woman who needed lots of help to lose weight. She had a stressful job and difficult home life with many family challenges. She also needed to work full-time to contribute to the household finances. The only respite from her stressful life came at lunchtime, when she dashed to her car and drove to a local coffee shop where she purchased her lunch, always a huge French baguette with luxurious fillings, accompanied by a large coffee. She sat and ate while reading a book. The two activities combined gave her some welcome relief from the other 23 hours in her day. The huge loaded sandwich also served to anaesthetize her from everything that was wrong with her life.

Behavior changes were urgently required. First, eat only half the baguette (it was huge). Same sandwich, same delicious fillings, but when you focus *only on the eating* you enjoy it as much as if it was the super-sized version. Then I asked, "Do you love reading?" She replied that she loved reading and it was her main pleasure in life. "Then why would you distract yourself from the pleasure of reading by eating your sandwich at the same time? You are doing two very pleasurable activities to relax you, to make you feel as if you've had a treat and to help you to face the rest of your working day. Why don't you *double* your enjoyment by doing them separately?" She couldn't fault my logic and went on to practice "eating less but enjoying it more" with her smaller-sized sandwich. Afterwards, she read her page-turner until the end of her lunch break, absorbed fully in the story. She discovered that this new, more pleasurable lunchtime helped her to deal with the stressful remainder of her day.

I offer this example to show how simple, achievable changes can make a dramatic difference to many aspects of your life. But there is another important aspect of this case. The life stress was the driver for over-eating. It was unbearable for her. She was in survival mode. It was clear this life would have to be healed in order for there to be lasting, sustainable weight loss. After many weeks of working hard with the program, her outlook had completely transformed. She was able to change everything about the way she used food to relieve the stress in her life. She learned how to relieve stress by using the superior, more effective techniques she had learned which included both guided meditations and acutapping techniques (simplified versions of these acutapping techniques are set out in Chapters 4 and 9).

She contacted me several years later to tell me how well she was continuing to do, and that she had never gone back to her old eating habits. She now had total control and could focus on making her life exactly how she wanted it to be. It's easy to look back and see how to change things for the better, but when you are inside that deep dark hole, solutions may be hidden from you, or you just don't have the energy to change things.

I didn't have a walking meditation in the program at that time. To design such a product and make it work requires the expertise of skilled sound engineers to add the exact frequencies to support the appropriate state of focused awareness, with your eyes open at all times to allow the walk to be navigated safely. If this walking meditation had been available, a lunchtime walk would have been incorporated into this woman's program, with wonderful benefits for her stress levels. The appropriate Hemi-Sync® frequencies encourage you to engage with the action of walking. You enjoy the meditative movement of your body as you adjust your pace, relax, breathe deeply and slow down your mind. You enjoy each moment. You let go of everyday stresses and worries, all the while absorbing the positive, supportive messages that will embed your slim, healthy goals deep into your mind. You will return from your walk refreshed, filled with a sense of wellbeing, ready for whatever comes next in your day.

This is multi-tasking on a superior level.

INHABIT EVERY PART OF YOURSELF AS YOU WALK

When I practiced this track and synchronized my breathing with my steps, I noticed something interesting. I could either walk to a regular pace, four beats in a bar, in what is called a "march" or "common" time in written music. Or if my pace was slower, my breathing automatically adjusted to three beats in a bar which is a "waltz." The waltzing pattern made for very interesting whole body relaxation. A sense of playfulness evolved. It was an interesting variation on regular, evenly-paced walking. You can experiment for yourself and find out what your body likes best.

When you walk, inhabit every part of your body. Notice your arms swinging by your sides and the feeling of your feet on the ground as you walk along. Be aware of the air around you, the coolness or warmth, the feeling of the breeze on your face and in your hair. Your eyes are alert and focused on your journey, making every adjustment for any changes of direction, obstacles, places where you should stop for traffic or pause to check your route. Notice the scent of your surroundings, the way the air smells. All the while, you are listening to the positive messages in your ears.

Keep your eyes level, unless you are navigating any obstacles or need to watch your step. This simple action has many positive benefits that are connected with the way your eye position is related to your emotional state. Keeping your eyes level or looking up at the sky from time to time will make your mood feel lighter. If you are a person who tends to look down when you walk about, you can try this simple tip and notice how it makes you feel.

If your habit is to use walking time to look at your phone, your eyes will be looking downwards as you do this. Notice other people who are also checking their phones as they walk along. It is estimated there is a postural catastrophe waiting to happen from all those bent necks and hunched shoulders that are ruining people's skeletal health all over the world. If you recognize yourself in this description, this walking meditation will be great for breaking your addiction to checking your phone as you walk. You may have to work at keeping your eyes level by giving yourself frequent reminders as you go along. It's a good, positive habit to get into. But watch out for those obstacles on your path. On the positive side, you'll notice and avoid all the lampposts, trees and road signs that you would otherwise have bumped into if your eyes had been fixed on your phone.

As you continue walking, keeping your eyes level or looking up from time to time, take in everything you see, scan your horizons and keep your mind focused on everything around you. Allow your vision to be drawn to things that give you pleasure or that interest you. Walking is a wonderful way to let go of all the stresses and strains of everyday life. A simple phrase to help you put your stresses into perspective is, "It's not what happens to you in life, but how you feel about it." I *know* you can easily change how you feel about things. All the techniques utilized in this album and the explanations in this book have the capability to improve the way you feel about things.

PUTTING YOURSELF FIRST

One of the themes in this program is that *it's okay to put yourself first*. In fact, to achieve the slim, healthy body you wish for, you will need to prioritize your own needs. Putting yourself at the bottom of your "to-do" list has most likely been a contributing factor in your weight gain or lack of dieting success in the past. Breaking free from your self-imposed rules about what has priority in your life will have unexpected benefits. You will be pleasantly surprised by how well this works in practice. Put your own health and wellbeing first, and amazingly your life does not fall apart. I guarantee it.

"Light and free, free to choose the life you want, free to choose to focus on your own goals, free to put your wishes and needs first. And of course, that's okay, because all your responsibilities, your commitments will still be honored. It's okay to put yourself first because you are important. Maybe many people depend on you. You need to be healthy and full of energy."

— *Walking Meditation,* Track 10

"But," you say, "but, but, I can't do it. I have too many responsibilities, I have too much on my plate, I have no time in my life, too many people depend on me." Don't worry, I *know* all of that to be true. Like many people in our super-fast world, I have experienced those same thoughts and feelings, as if you are a hamster on a wheel and cannot get off. However, I challenge you to consider how much use you are to the many people who depend on you, at home and at work, if you are overweight, unhealthy, exhausted, and your "get up and go" has got up and gone.

A central part of this program is to take you (kicking and screaming, if necessary) and place you at the top of your list of priorities. This is not a joke. This is serious business. There is no "get out of jail free" card for your health and wellbeing. If you do not put yourself first then your ability to discharge your responsibilities will falter and fail. You may become ill. I assure you, your mind (whose job it is to protect you) is perfectly capable of making you ill to slow you down and force you to get off that treadmill. I know how busy and stressed you may be. That is why this walking meditation has been designed to be a triumph of multi-tasking. By using it, you are getting the most out of a thrifty 20 minutes of your precious day. This time spent walking and meditating will do you more good than many hours of unfocused relaxation in front of the TV or whatever is your usual mode of winding down.

Perhaps you never get any time to wind down. Perhaps you flop into bed still hyped-up from an evening of relentless activity. I urge you to make using this meditation a priority. You are not skimping on any other of your important responsibilities and you are gaining wonderful benefits.

It may take a few weeks before you finally absorb the message to prioritize your own health and welfare, a message that is woven into many of the tracks. However, every day you will add a layer of loving self-care into your routine, perhaps without you even realizing it.

YOUR LIST OF PRIORITIES

Before we move on, I'd like you to make a list of all the people (or creatures or inanimate objects) that come before you in importance in your life. These are the people, creatures or things that take priority over you. All their needs, no matter how unreasonable, must be satisfied before you can have what you need. Be honest! If the list you make contains sensitive information you have permission to shred it afterwards or destroy it in some way.

The following list includes many of the answers I have received from people when I asked this question. Rearrange the order, as necessary:

- Children.
- Dog or other pet.
- Work.
- Having a new kitchen.
- Husband/wife/partner.
- Profile on social media.
- Best friend.
- Doing your overdue taxes.

- The number of calories in a margarita.
- Where your teenager was last Thursday.
- Your collection of tropical fish.
- The leaking bathroom tap.
- Where you can find a good plumber.
- The state of the world.
- The state of your yard.
- The car and how to explain that dent in the bumper.
- Cleaning out the garage.
- Your own health and welfare.

What will it take for you to insert your own health and welfare at the top of the list and to prioritize your journey to a slim, healthy body? This album with all its positive messages will do 90% of the work, but you must make a firm decision to take that final 10% step. You are not selfish. You will not become spoiled or unlikable. All that will happen is you will energize your journey and everyone else will benefit. The people in your life may even comment about how much more you are doing for them, how much they feel your love and care and your appreciation. Everyone is a winner. And you will find a good plumber, I promise!

THIS WALKING MEDITATION SUMMARIZES THE MAIN THEMES

When you start this program, you are advised to concentrate fully on doing the meditations and to follow the eating instructions to the letter. By using the meditations every single day (you can vary the tracks, depending on what you need), you will be working at a deep level to support yourself emotionally and psychologically. You will be building up your inner strength and building your resilience to allow you to cope with whatever life throws at you. By using meditations every day and finding time to incorporate them into your schedule, you increase your progress rate exponentially. This *Walking Meditation* summarizes "eating less but enjoying it more." It is your opportunity to remind yourself about how you are going to change the way you eat and lose all of your unwanted weight. This walking meditation takes about 20 minutes. It will give you all the benefits of exercise and relaxation while building up your inner resources. You will therefore put the work in and get the results out.

THE BENEFITS OF MEDITATION

Meditation reduces your stress levels and this effect will be greatly enhanced by enjoying a refreshing walk. Your base rate of stress reduces each time you meditate. After a week or two, a sense of relaxation that is physical, mental and emotional becomes your norm. When you feel relaxed, even difficult life challenges are easier to cope with. When you approach life with a clear head, obstacles that used to get in your way simply dissolve. Your mind, freed from constantly thinking about food, can use its intelligence to come up with creative ways to optimize everything about your life.

Over many years I have worked with people who have become overweight due to stress, overwork and lifestyle challenges. This program fixes all of that *from the inside out*. While you may not yet believe it's possible, I challenge you to work at your meditation tracks and notice the changes in your life.

When you work regularly with guided meditations, your mind will slow down. The act of meditating in this prescribed format, with the Hemi-Sync® frequencies in the background, will slow down the speed of your thoughts and allow you to focus more fully in what you are doing. Therefore, whatever you do will then have your full attention. You will not be distracted by a myriad of competing thoughts, diverting your attention from the task in hand. You become more efficient. You may become super-efficient. You can do more with less time, simply by learning how to slow your mind down so you have all your attention in one place where you need it. If you want to become super-efficient, give this program 100% of your energy and do it exactly as prescribed.

MULTI-TASKING DO'S AND DON'TS

I am a big fan of multi-tasking when it's applied to doing what needs to be done while listening to guided meditations at the same time. This walking meditation is designed for multi-tasking. The track of *Affirmations for a Slim, Healthy Body* is also perfect for listening to and repeating out loud when you are doing something else. There are some practical limitations; you must not use meditations while you are driving or doing any task which may result in a safety risk to yourself or others.

But have you considered doing your emails (or any other computer-based activity which is necessary, repetitive and potentially stressful) while listening to a track from this album? You turn the volume down a bit so your conscious mind can focus fully on your emails while your subconscious mind can absorb more positive messages from the meditation. I have used this technique many times over the years and it works beautifully. It's interesting to notice how, by the end of the track, you have cleared your email backlog but your breathing is deep and relaxed, your mind is sharp and you feel energized. If you do your emails as normal, your body becomes tense, your mind overloaded and you feel drained. To me that is enough motivation to give this meditation-based multi-tasking idea a thorough trial. It also works well with repetitive tasks that you already do without much conscious thought, like household chores, gardening, walking the dog or going around the supermarket.

Take a moment to think about times when you could add in some extra practice to enhance your experience. Everyone will think you are listening to your music playlist, but you'll know better.

One of my first clients was a lady who suffered from claustrophobia. When she explained the severity of her symptoms, I was shocked. I wondered how she had found the courage to get out of her home and come to my practice. Every closed-in space gave her appalling physical anxiety. The feeling of the bedclothes on her body scared her. A cloudy sky made her feel panicky as if the sky was closing in on her. She could not drive without having the car windows fully open. I wrote a hypnotherapy treatment specifically for her and recorded it. She also took home my basic relaxation track to mix in and give her some variety in her homework.

This lady was a model client, working hard at her meditation practice. I was impressed with her motivation. After several weeks, a smile began to appear on her face. She looked lighter, more energetic, less fearful. She explained she had established a routine with her hypnotherapy meditations. She told me she liked to hear my voice when she was in the house because it reassured her. In fact, she put the tracks on when she was doing her housework, her ironing, her vacuuming. She liked to turn the volume up really loud so she could hear my voice in all parts of the house. She was listening for many hours a day, soaking her mind with positive therapy.

I worried all the residents in the street would also be hearing the meditations, but reasoned everyone would benefit from the positive messages. Within a short time, this lady was fully recovered, she could face her life free from fear. I also learned something important. When you *immerse* yourself in these powerful techniques you can quickly make positive changes that you would never have thought possible.

HONOR THE EARTH'S BOUNTY

As you walk along listening to this meditation, outside, away from your indoor environment, you are encouraged to consider the relationship between this planet and the food that is earth's bounty. For many of us, food is something to be purchased in a brightly-lit supermarket. Each item will be packed in sterile, plastic wrapping and washed clean of all traces of where the food came from. It is good, therefore, to turn your attention to the origins of the foods you love to eat, tracing their provenance back to the soil, the air, the clean water and the energy from the sun. This part of the track is to help you link what you love to eat now with where the food comes from in its purest form. Take a moment to be grateful for everything that has been provided for us here in this "Garden of Eden."

"You notice the foods you love to eat are foods that contain the goodness of earth's bounty, the sunshine and rain, the harvest of nourishment that our planet provides for us. Take a moment to honor and respect all aspects of this wonderful harvest, and all those who contribute to its production."

— Walking Meditation, Track 10

Make an effort to mentally connect to all those people whose life's work is connected with growing and nurturing food from all sources. Your imagination will supply you with images and ideas to work with. You may focus on something you really enjoy eating. Allow your mind to think about all the stages of growth and production from field to your plate. Send thanks to all who are involved in your enjoyment. Send thanks to the earth.

Increasing your awareness of this connection will strengthen your understanding of how important it is to provide your body with nourishing food. I am confident that by eating, tasting and enjoying food properly, your desire for good food will grow and your taste for all things processed will reduce. When you are listening to the track and hear the suggestion to connect with an image of earth's bounty, I doubt that the image will be a factory with complex processes that use lots of chemicals.

Your awareness will evolve as you continue to listen to what your body is telling you to eat, tasting your food fully, and then noticing how your body, mind and emotions react to what you eat. You will be the one in charge of this evolution of your food preferences. You can make your own decisions about what is good for you and what doesn't suit you.

MODERN ATTITUDES TO FOOD

Some people hold extreme opinions about food. In the last 50 years or so, we have been encouraged (by scientists, medical professionals, experts, dieticians and the media) to label foods as "good" or "bad." Current research continues to delve deeper into what happens to food inside our bodies, and then link consumption of these foods to certain diseases. The resultant reports always make headline news.

Turn back the clock to before industrialization and many "bad" foods were considered staple foods. Bread, butter, milk, cheese, meat, fish and eggs, supplemented by vegetables and fruits in season, were the foundations of a healthy, balanced diet. How many of these foods are now excluded from people's diets because of fashion or food trends?

One hundred and fifty years ago, in the new industrialized cities of the UK, drinking water from communal wells or pumps was likely to give you a serious illness. *Beer* was therefore a staple drink to avoid serious diseases such as cholera or typhoid. Children drank "small beer," small cups of beer with a lower alcohol strength. Can you imagine the outrage if you regularly gave your child beer to drink? You'd be arrested! Yet this practice saved young lives and was appropriate at the time.

Before refrigeration, it was important to preserve foods when there was a glut at harvest time, so sweet preserves were made, fruit was dried and bottled, honey was collected and put into jars. Meat and fish were preserved with salt and smoking. Milk was made into cheese. Vegetables and fruits were canned or pickled to accompany bland winter meals and make them more interesting. Beans were dried for cooking later on the year. Nothing was wasted because otherwise you were likely to go hungry. Yet many of these nourishing foods are now rejected as unhealthy. Humankind survived eating foods that do not pass the modern test about what is healthy or unhealthy, good or bad. People survived and thrived despite the health challenges which include no antibiotics, vaccinations, anesthetics, surgery, clean water and safe sewage disposal. People also survived during times when food was very scarce and you had to eat anything you could get your hands on.

If you have absorbed strong beliefs about food from all sources of media, your attitudes may be set firm about what are good foods and bad foods. If your diet is composed only of foods you think are "clean" or "healthy" or "full of antioxidants" or "containing 75% of your RDA of omega 3", then I urge you to *relax* about your food. Think about your ancestors. Imagine the kinds of meals your parents and grandparents ate. Remember the meals you experienced in the past, before you believed what the so-called experts told you. Ask yourself this: "What should I believe about what is good for me? My own body, or the findings of some scientific report or the tweets of a famous social media influencer?" You know yourself best. Always remember that.

COMPLETING YOUR WALK
As you complete your walk, your mind will be reaffirming all the important suggestions for you to progress on your journey towards a slim, healthy body. Your footsteps are a metaphor for the journey. Your mind will be refreshed and your willpower will be boosted. You will get through your day with more zing.

I hope you find it easy and enjoyable to incorporate this walking meditation into your routine. I know there will be many, many benefits from doing it. Walking is the exact opposite of sitting hunched over your desk, or rushing around doing chores, or dashing from place to place in your car, or slumping in front of the TV for a little rest. And that, in itself, must be a good thing.

CHAPTER 11
AFFIRMATIONS FOR A SLIM, HEALTHY BODY

"Affirmations support your journey towards a slim, healthy future by reminding you of the key elements of success. Listen while in your ordinary waking consciousness. Repeat these phrases out loud or to yourself and they will form a deep and lasting impression."
— *Affirmations for a Slim, Healthy Body,* Track 11

This track is designed to be used while doing everyday activities. The phrases and the background music with Hemi-Sync® frequencies will not lead you into a deeper state where you may lose awareness. When you engage with the affirmations by repeating them aloud, or quietly inside, you are keeping your mind in the now, concentrating on whatever other task you are doing.

Affirmations are best used when doing other repetitive activities that do not require your full attention. Any physical activity that really does need your full concentration, such as driving or using machinery, or where you could hurt yourself if you became absorbed in the verbal guidance, is not a suitable complement for affirmations. This advice also applies to times when you may be responsible for the safety of others. Therefore, use your own judgment about how to fit in these affirmations into your everyday life.

AFFIRMATIONS CAN FILL IN THE SPACES IN YOUR LIFE

Life has many periods of unproductive downtime. Waiting for an expected phone call or appointment. Collecting children from after-school activities. Waiting for an important package to be delivered. Waiting for your computer to configure after those annoying updates. Waiting for a friend to call, the bathroom to be free, the kettle to boil, the dinner to be ready. Modern life is full of waiting time. Affirmations are a great way to fill that time.

Many happy hours of listening can be included while you prepare dinner — *while you prepare dinner*. Not while you wait for the takeout to be delivered, or the microwave to ping. Making food for yourself and those you care about is an affirmation all by itself. You affirm your commitment to eating delicious food and getting the maximum pleasure out of it. If you have a pile of veggies to chop up, affirmations can make this task a revelation of calm and enjoyment. I like carrots but, boy, can chopping carrots make you feel tense. Chop, chop, chop. Slicing stir-fry vegetables into small dice is another stress-making task that seems to go on forever. Listening and repeating the affirmations will slow your breathing and focus your attention on your goals. Be careful with that knife!

If you enjoy any kind of creative activity, you can use this time to do your affirmations. You may already listen to music while you paint or draw or knit or make model trains or dresses or re-pot your geraniums. Affirmations can make those special relaxation times very productive. The benefits of listening to these tracks have already been explored in the previous chapter, *Walking Meditation*. When you listen in the waking state, there is a specific feeling of awareness that you experience. It seems like you are fully in the "now," neither fretting about the things that happened during the day nor worrying about what you will be doing later. You can enjoy that state of awareness, secure in the knowledge that your mind will absorb the positive affirmations and your tasks will be completed perfectly.

You do not need peace and quiet. You do not need to speak the phrases aloud if it's not convenient for you. Silent repetition in your head is just fine.

This album contains 12 tracks to choose from to make this journey towards a slim, healthy body a success. Therefore, if you prefer to sit back and listen to a different track, go ahead. There is something for every mood. You may choose these affirmations as an easy way to deepen your resolve when you have short periods of time to fill. No imagination or visualization or focus is required. It doesn't matter what state of mind you are in when you start. By the end you'll be in your own zone of calm, with the positive phrases ringing in your ears.

CONSTRUCTION OF THE AFFIRMATIONS
The affirmations I have chosen are based on the positive messages that are explored during the tracks. They are expressions of willpower. When you say them to yourself, your mind absorbs the statements and stores them so it can feed them back to you at the appropriate time when you might need to hear them. There are many phrases, based on what people have told me when I asked the question: "Tell me 10 things that are going to stop you reaching your weight loss goal?" By turning the resulting answers into the *positive*, affirmations are created.

You may notice the phrases are short and expressed in the first person. In my experience, that is how the mind generally speaks to you. It doesn't start telling you a long, convoluted story when you stand in front of the refrigerator, looking for something to pop into your mouth. I simply says, "I can't be bothered to diet today," or "I'm too tired to make dinner," or "I'll start again tomorrow." And because the phrases are relatively generic, there is plenty of room for you to personalize them. By taking some time to fine-tune these affirmations into your own exact words you will make them even more powerful.

Read through the list and pick out the 10 most important affirmations that sum up your own challenges. You can then rewrite them in the same short, punchy style to make them your own. Commit them to paper and keep them nearby for reference, or you can record them on your phone. Your own voice will carry a lot of power and ensure you take these affirmations to heart.

1. I am determined to slim down to my goal weight.
2. Nothing is going to stop me.
3. I am confident and focused.
4. I have iron willpower, I will succeed.
5. I love to plan my meals for maximum enjoyment.
6. I enjoy giving myself good food to eat.
7. My stomach is about the size of a large orange.
8. That's the right amount of food for me to eat.
9. I eat only at mealtimes so I can appreciate my food.
10. I eat less but enjoy it more — I never feel deprived.
11. I listen carefully to what my body wants.
12. I give myself enough time to enjoy my food properly.
13. Food tastes great when I focus on what I'm eating.
14. I choose to be peaceful and quiet when I'm eating.
15. At the end of each meal I feel full and satisfied.
16. I make every meal a special occasion.
17. I make getting slim my top priority.
18. My health and vitality are important.
19. I know I can succeed if I stick to my plan.
20. I feel full of energy and I radiate good health.
21. Every morning I feel slimmer and more healthy.
22. I look forward to enjoying my food every day.
23. Being organized is my way to ensure success.

24. I look forward to being a little slimmer every day.
25. The time in between meals are my favorite times of day.
26. Every day I can enrich my life with new exciting things to do.
27. Exercise is my way of making myself feel fitter and stronger.
28. I enjoy trying new activities that make me feel alive.
29. When I try something new, I feel my confidence grow.
30. My body appreciates all the attention I give it.
31. When I'm active, I am raising my metabolism.
32. My body responds by being more toned.
33. When I eat out, I feel completely in control.
34. I make wise but delicious choices when I eat out .
35. Eating out is all about the occasion and having fun.
36. I enjoy my temptation foods in moderation.
37. Food no longer has power over me.
38. My favorite foods are enjoyable in small amounts.
39. I am polite but firm when others try to make me eat more.
40. I prefer to have small delicious meals.
41. In social situations, I feel no pressure to overeat.
42. I simply eat less but enjoy it more.
43. I choose relaxation to deal with life's everyday pressures.
44. I no longer use food to cope with stressful situations.
45. I face my challenges head on by being calm and relaxed.
46. Things that used to bother me in the past no longer have the power to hurt me.
47. People and situations that hinder me — I just let go of them.
48. Everybody notices how much more happy and confident I am.
49. I deserve to be slim because I work hard at it.
50. I give myself regular messages of support.
51. I praise myself every day for the good job I'm doing.
52. I reinforce my self-worth with regular compliments.
53. When I stumble, I pick myself right up.
54. Life's challenges teach me how to be strong and determined.
55. And I like and respect myself, inside and out.
56. I am worthy of love and attention.

57. I allow my inner self to shine.
58. Life is good and I feel great.
59. As I reveal my slim, healthy body I grow in confidence.
60. Every step I take will guide me to my slim, healthy future.

This track of affirmations is a simple expression of everything you need to support you on this journey. I hope you find out how powerful these positive phrases are when they are incorporated into your own internal dialogue.

CHAPTER 12
SLIM AND HEALTHY FOR LIFE

"Welcome to *Slim and Healthy for Life*, the final Hemi-Sync® track on your journey into your slim, healthy future. This track is designed to ensure your long term success by working on that most important of skills — persevering onwards to your goal and never looking back. This is your guarantee of success. Those who succeed are those who never give up, no matter what."

— *Slim and Healthy for Life*, Track 12

You are reaching the final stage of your journey. At this point you will have learned everything required about making a slim, healthy future your reality *now*. All the meditation and acutapping resources you have used are still available to you. You will know when you need them. But now it's time to bring all the various elements together into one final meditation that will take you forward and guide you effortlessly as you enjoy everything about being slim and healthy.

This track focuses on persevering and never giving up. The suggestion of perseverance is embedded throughout the verbal guidance. There are also gentle reminders of other parts of the program, summarized so you can keep the important lessons that you have learned close to your consciousness and incorporate them into your everyday behavior. The track will serve to keep you moving as an unstoppable force towards that future that you imagined and energized in Track 7, *Overcoming Obstacles*.

Your wise inner self, your companion on this journey, joins you. You are encouraged to sense that you and your wise inner self are now one being. You are wise. You are transformed. You live your life as your wise inner self. As part of the guided relaxation at the start of the track, I ask you to summon a glow of colored light to spread out from your center and inhabit every part of you. This is the signal for you and your wise inner self to become one. Colored light can also have spiritual associations. Many people are able to "see" the light of auras, the electromagnetic field that radiates out from our bodies. The colors and patterns of the aura reflect the emotional and spiritual energy of the person. Therefore, at this point in the track, open your mind to whatever color your wise inner self shows you. Then work with it. Release any ideas about what the color might mean. All you need to know is that it's right for you at this time. Your color might change each time you listen to this track. Be curious to find out when this will happen and how it will make you feel.

> "Your willpower is like a sleeping dragon in your spine, resting easily but ready to roar when you need it. Enjoy a sense of that power inside..."
> — *Slim and Healthy for Life*, Track 12

Your willpower now spreads out into other areas of your life. The six skills that represent that personal power inside you:

1. *Determination:* You are completely determined in everything you do. You achieve your goals.
2. *Motivation:* The energy of your *incentive* to make life changes. You can imagine positive changes in your future and this makes you feel inspired to achieve them.

3. *Confidence:* You trust your abilities, you feel self-assured. You can do it!
4. *Focus:* You have total clarity about your goal. All your attention, your energy and your resources are concentrated on whatever you want to manifest in your life.
5. *Tenacity:* Stubborn and persistent, you stick to your goal, never giving up, no matter what difficulties come your way.
6. *Mental toughness:* You've made up your mind and that is it! Mentally resolute and intractable, strong and resilient, you hold firmly to your goal.

These skills are now available for you to use whenever you wish. It is your choice and you have total control. That is the wonder of working with your inner power. You can have control over your thoughts, emotions and behaviors. You can be flexible about when you choose to use your willpower skills to drive your life towards a specific goal, or simply let your life unfold in a relaxed, harmonious way. You will know when iron willpower is required! There will always be times when you want to be soft and yielding, taking life as it comes. Your sleeping dragon of willpower can remain asleep if you want it to.

MAINTAINING YOUR METABOLISM

You will then revisit the theme of the *Metabolism Boost* meditation to remind yourself of the imagery and the work you have done to optimize the rate at which you burn calories. You now have a vibrant furnace of cellular energy at your disposal. You remind yourself that your body now co-operates with you to work towards your goal.

You may have used the *Metabolism Boost* track to give you the energy and focus to become active. This is the way to keep your energy burning and promote good health while you do it. If you have ever read about people who have lost weight and changed their lives, they report that activity is now an important and enjoyable part of their schedule. And as the proud owner of a slim, healthy body you will be keen to make full use of it by being active. When you do so, you'll be honoring the work you have put in. Why would you want to go back to the old ways of living? This body of yours deserves to be shown off proudly. There are many pleasurable ways to enjoy activity, both inside and outside in the fresh air. Activity will enhance your life. Try as many kinds of activity as you can fit in to your schedule. Be inquisitive about what different activities are like. Sometimes it's not about the activity but the people you meet when you do it. New horizons await!

THE PAST IS NOW RESOLVED

You are reminded about how you dissolved the hurts from the past. You only need a gentle reminder of your previous work using the *Release the Past* meditation, because your mind will have a clear record of everything you've done to resolve issues that were holding you back. It will only take a moment for your mind to register and note this gentle reminder.

"You now have mastery of your thoughts. Your heightened insight into your mind and emotions creates an atmosphere of positive energy."
— *Slim and Healthy for Life,* Track 12

Resolving past hurts is another way to gain control of your thoughts and emotions in the present. When the past is resolved, there is no reason for you to be burdened with the reminders of what happened in the past. By bringing your memories up to conscious awareness and by healing those memories, you neutralize all the negative emotional energy from those past events. Therefore, you now have choices about what to think and feel, as opposed to receiving constant mental reminders about past events that you cannot change.

LIFE HAS MANY OBSTACLES TO OVERCOME

We are not in charge of the challenges that life throws at us. We only have control over how we *think* and *feel* about them. When you are in control of your thoughts and in harmony with your emotions, you will be able to remain calm and do whatever is necessary to get yourself through to the other side. You will also be a shining example to others about how to navigate through the challenges, and make the best and wisest decisions. People always make better decisions when they are calm.

"You have a light touch. You can find ways to navigate around all the obstacles you may face with grace and elegance."
— *Slim and Healthy for Life,* Track 12

You are next reminded about the track for overcoming obstacles. Again, your mind will make instant links to all the times you worked with the track, and all the insight and inner resources you gained. Obstacles come in many shapes and sizes. They may appear to be insurmountable, but when you work with them using your powerful imagination, you can reveal exactly what your obstacles represent and how you can overcome them. The process will work even if you don't know what the obstacle is. Sometimes you may feel as if you have a mental block about something. You can't put your finger on what is wrong, therefore you can't begin to solve the problem. At other times you may feel as if you are in a fog and cannot see what you should do. In both cases, the block and the fog can be used as your obstacle in Track 7.

You may find that using this final track will pinpoint an issue that requires you to go back and work on the main *Overcoming Obstacles* track to help solve the issue. This is not a step backwards, but merely a recognition that you want to be thorough in working through every aspect of your journey towards a slim, healthy future.

A POSITIVE AND HARMONIOUS RELATIONSHIP WITH FOOD
Right from the start, you learned that food must assume its rightful place in your life. Food is a natural source of pleasure and enjoyment, nourishment and comfort and will continue to be so. Across the world,

in all different cultures and societies, happy events and celebrations are accompanied by delicious food. You have gained a vital understanding about food that will ensure you go forward in your life with food as your friend. Delicious food of all kinds has an important role to play in your slim, healthy future life. That is exactly as it should be.

Whatever kind of relationship you had with food when you began, by working diligently with the tracks you will have established a respectful, loving and harmonious relationship with your food. The practical aspects of eating less but enjoying it more have encouraged you to let go of all unhelpful attitudes to food. You may have been convinced that many foods were bad or would cause disease. You may have had an optimistic view of the health benefits of certain foods. You may have been scared of food. Or angry with the way food had made you put on weight. You may have been obsessed with food and thought about nothing else all day long.

None of these relationships with food is respectful or loving or harmonious. Therefore, at this stage in the track, there is a gentle reminder to reaffirm that food is now in its rightful place. It doesn't have power over you. You can be free from all aspects of negative thinking and emotions concerning food.

"Food and eating are no longer the center of your world. Your world is so much bigger and more exciting than that."
— *Slim and Healthy for Life,* Track 12

ACTIVITY IS PART OF YOUR SLIM FUTURE

Your metabolism is boosted by inner work and physical activity. The next short section reminds you about the many wonderful activities you can choose from. If I asked you to investigate all the sports and activities that people enjoy, I would estimate the resulting list would contain hundreds of choices. Humans love to be active. But when you have been hiding inside a body that you weren't proud of, it may take courage to get out there in the world and become more active.

There is a well-known TV series that promotes a 12-month program for very seriously overweight people. The candidates are nominated by relatives and then are chosen to take part in a diet and exercise transformation. Every effort goes into supporting them with their weight loss and activity program. Sometimes psychological therapies are employed. Yet, if you have watched this program, you'll know that much of the exercise consists of punishing gym routines done in the person's own home. Often the living space has a home gym installed as part of the show. We witness the person engaged in brutal workouts to get to their goal weight.

Does that idea put your off being active? Does exercise have to be *brutal* and *punishing* to be effective? Do we even like those words? Or do they remind you of the other ways we speak about diets and weight loss? For example: "battle of the bulge" or "fighting the flab" (both UK catch phrases) or "struggling to lose weight" or "crash diet" — all of which make losing weight sound difficult and unappealing.

Where are the words of gentle encouragement? Where are the words that speak of enjoyment and pleasure and something wonderful to look forward to? By this time you already know that the journey towards your slim, healthy future has been an exploration of the joys and pleasures of life. Relentlessly positive. Exploring all the ways you can have more fun. Therefore, activity must also be fun. I forbid you from doing any activity that does not make you feel good!

If you decide to make a list of activities you want to try out, make sure you will gain pleasure and enjoyment from each one. Did you enjoy the *Walking Meditation*, walking for 20 minutes, taking in everything around you, looking up and experiencing your environment using all your senses? Sometimes simple physical activity is the most fun.

Whatever activities you decide on to be more active in your slim body, make sure they are what *you* want to do. You may feel pressured by friends or family or you may be influenced by other role models in the public eye. Think of yourself as an individual with your personal likes and dislikes. Do not be swayed by those who think that you have to experience pain in order to gain benefits from an active lifestyle.

CHOOSING POSITIVE LIFE CHANGES

After the reminders of the key points from different tracks on the album, there comes a section for you to work interactively on making a positive change in your life. This can be anything connected with any part of your life.

You have already explored a slim future in the *Overcoming Obstacles* track, enjoying the feeling of inhabiting a slim body. Now it is time to take that exploration one step further and consider positive life changes that are connected with your future slim self.

For a few minutes, while you enjoy the Hemi-Sync® frequencies in the background, take yourself into the future and use your imagination to explore one positive change you want to make in your life. You can make this a small change or a big change. We know your imagination has the capability to add power and energy to whatever you want to work on. You can rehearse your chosen positive change and by doing so, send a message to your whole self, body, mind and spirit, that you want this change to happen.

You can start small. Think about an example of wanting to drink more water in your work life. You may work in a place that is air-conditioned and stuffy. You get dehydrated. Yet you keep forgetting to drink or you don't like the taste of the water available or you don't have the right water container. Take a few minutes during this track to explore being at work with the proper water container, filled with the water you prefer, flavored or not. Picture yourself drinking and staying hydrated. Notice how you feel at the end of the day. Then use the images to change your drinking habits.

Another example: You intend to walk more and use your walking meditation, but things get in your way. Lunch breaks seem so short. You struggle to leave the office. You cave in to pressure to keep on working. At the end of the day you want to get home as quickly as possible. A walk is the last thing you want to do. Choose this intended change to work on during the meditation. Explore what you have to say and do at work to find that time to walk during your lunch break. Practice saying the words that will make it happen. Imagine writing your walk in your schedule, either your diary or in whatever computer program you use at work. Then imagine enjoying the walk. Imagine the wonderful sense of outdoors. Imagine different kinds of weather. Plan for how to enjoy your walk whatever the weather. Walking in the rain is empowering, but you need to plan to have dry clothes available if you need them.

A final example: A big life change. You want to try something new in your life, such as leaving your career to train for a different work life, or maybe to travel around the world. You'll need confidence and resources. Use this time during the track to explore the main elements of this change. Focus on the imagery of having achieved your goal.

Interestingly, your mind is fully capable of instantly providing you with the information about the steps you have to take to get there. You'll gain insight. You can explore how you feel.

If you have big dreams, and if you want to work on making them real using guided meditations, the Hemi-Sync® title *Creating a Positive Future* is recommended. It's a complete manifesting track suitable for using to make your big life dreams come true.

AFFIRMATIONS ARE ALWAYS A GOOD WAY TO FINISH

I hope by now you are a fan of affirmations. Simple in construction but powerful in practice, these targeted phrases are designed to be integrated into your inner dialogue.

You may have already designed some positive phrases that are unique to you. You may have recorded them on your device to remind you of your goals. Creating affirmations requires you to listen to your own inner words, the way in which your mind speaks to you, often including negative and self-defeating language. You then turn the words around to make a positive and inspiring "antidote" which becomes your affirmation. There are some simple rules to be followed. Always write affirmations in the first person and make them short and snappy. Use words that are part of your normal vocabulary. Then look at what you have written and check to see if you can add something to make the phrases more compelling, more appealing. An affirmation your mind will not want to resist. Add in some words that have a "pull."

If you want your affirmation to say something like, "I stay out of the refrigerator in case I am tempted to eat a snack," notice how that expression sounds a little negative and uninteresting. Make it more appealing by saying, "I surprise myself with how easy it is to resist what's in the refrigerator," or you may prefer "I am filled with willpower and I am immune to snacking."

As you go forward into your slim future, you will become self-reliant. You'll be your own therapist who knows exactly which areas of your life you need to pay attention to. You may be curious to find out how to take the next steps on your journey of self-discovery. As mentioned previously, the Hemi-Sync® website will inspire you with its many products to take you in whatever direction you want to explore.

But perhaps, just perhaps, your slim future will become a time for you to relax into your life and enjoy the flow. It's not always necessary to be pushing or progressing all the time. Life is meant to be enjoyable, and you now have permission to go ahead and find that joy. And as you go about your daily life, you might inspire others who would benefit from taking control of their own lives and circumstances. You will not have to say or do anything. It will seem as if something inside you is shining out and touching the hearts and minds of others who may also want to change. Everything that you have achieved, all your inner work and all the effort you have put into this journey, will create a positive force that is unconsciously visible to those around you. By changing your-self, you have the potential to inspire others to change. And that is a wonderful thing.

ABOUT HEMI-SYNC®

Hemi-Sync® frequencies provide the foundation for change during your journey towards a slim, healthy body. For those who are new to verbally-guided meditations and have no prior understanding about Hemi-Sync® audio technology, it's useful to gain insights into the background and the many benefits that will support your own journey towards a slim, healthy body. When you listen to the 12 guided meditations, you will engage with the powerful messages in the tracks, but the music and audio tones, with their specific sound patterns and frequencies, support the messages in a unique way.

The following information which is taken from the Hemi-Sync® website, explains exactly how the accompanying music, and the pink sound patterns featured in many of the tracks, are an integral part of the program.

Robert A. Monroe, founder of Hemi-Sync®, is internationally known for his work with audio sound patterns that can have dramatic effects on states of consciousness. Monroe observed, during his early research, that certain sounds create a *Frequency Following Response* in the electrical activity of the brain. Those observations led to some remarkable findings dealing with the very nature of human consciousness. Researchers learned specific sounds could be blended and sequenced to gently lead the brain to various states ranging from deep relaxation or sleep to expanded states of awareness and other extraordinary states. This compelling research became the foundation of a non-invasive and easy-to-use audio-guidance technology known as Hemi-Sync®.

The audio guidance process works through the generation of complex, multi-layered audio signals. Signals act together to create a resonance that is reflected in unique brainwave forms characteristic of specific states of consciousness. The result is a focused whole brain state called hemispheric synchronization or Hemi-Sync®, where the left and right hemispheres are working together in a state of coherence. Different Hemi-Sync® signals are used to facilitate deep relaxation, focused attention or other desired states. As an analogy, lasers produce focused, coherent light. Hemi-Sync® produces a focused coherent mind, which is an optimal condition for producing improved human performance.

One of the leading researchers into brain wave synchrony, Dr. Lester Fehmi, of the Princeton Biofeedback Research Institute, points out that "Synchrony represents the maximum efficiency of information transport through the whole brain." This means that brainwave synchrony produces a sharp increase in the effects of various brain wave states. The production of synchronized, coherent electro-magnetic energy by the human brain at a given frequency leads to a 'laser-like' condition increasing the amplitude and strength of the brainwaves. It's evident that a "highly integrated brain," a brain, in which both hemispheres are functioning in symmetry, synchrony, harmony and unity, is a key to peak states and peak human performance.

Specific combinations of Hemi-Sync® signals, for example, can help individuals achieve laser-like focus and concentration. Depending on the intended goals, music, verbal guidance or subtle sound effects are combined with Hemi-Sync® to strengthen its effectiveness. Naturally, Hemi-Sync® sleep products incorporate predominately Delta frequencies; learning products predominantly Beta, and so forth.

Users remain in total control as these recordings do not contain subliminal messages. Hemispheric synchronization does occur naturally in daily life, but typically only for random, brief periods of time. Hemi-Sync® can assist individuals in achieving and sustaining this highly productive, coherent, brain wave state.

Robert Monroe's work inspired an entire industry of mind/brain products. After more than 50 years of research, and thousands of lab sessions, the internationally acclaimed patented Hemi-Sync® process remains unparalleled in its ability to assist us in harnessing our human potential.

Thanks to the cooperation of notable medical institutions and universities, the scientifically and clinically proven Hemi-Sync® technology continues to be the focus of a variety of specialized research projects. In addition, many therapists, physicians, educators, and other professionals use Hemi-Sync® extensively.

Such research is indispensable in revealing the influence of specific Hemi-Sync® sound patterns on consciousness. Over the years, these efforts have resulted in the development of scores of individual products for specific applications such as focused attention, stress management, meditation, sleep enhancement, and pain management, to name a few.

WHAT DOES THIS MEAN FOR YOU?
Hemi-Sync® can help you experience enhanced mental, physical, and emotional states, by combining verbal guidance, music, pink sound and/or other audio effects with the binaural beats. The particular elements for each recording are carefully selected and integrated with

the appropriate Hemi-Sync® sound frequencies to enhance the desired effect.

IT ALL HAPPENS IN THE BRAIN

The brain controls all body activities, ranging from heart rate and breathing to emotion, learning, and memory. It is even thought to influence the immune system's response to disease. It sets humans apart from all other species by allowing us to achieve scientific breakthroughs, composing masterpieces of literature, art, and music. The brain is what makes us human. The extent of the brain's capabilities is unknown; it is the most complex living structure known in the universe

The brain is divided into two hemispheres — left and right. The left hemisphere has been linked with verbal skills, rational, logical, and analytical thinking. The right hemisphere has been linked with visual/spatial skills, emotion, musical aptitude, intuition, and imaginative thought. There is a reason why we have two hemispheres: they are both necessary and complementary, and they function best when they are functioning together. It is well known that the brain is an electrochemical organ; researchers have speculated that a fully functioning brain can generate as much as 10 watts of electrical power. Even though this electrical power is very limited, it does occur in very specific ways that are characteristic of the human brain. Electrical activity emanating from the brain is displayed in the form of brain waves.

Beta brain waves are the fastest frequencies ranging from 14 cycles per second up to 38 cycles per second. Beta is your normal thinking state, your active external awareness and thought process. Without Beta you would not be able to function in the outside world.

Alpha brain waves are the brain waves of relaxed detached awareness, visualization, sensory imagery and light reverie. Ranging between about 9 cycles per second and 14 cycles per second, Alpha is the gateway to meditation and provides a bridge between the conscious and the subconscious mind.

Theta brainwaves are the subconscious mind. Ranging from about 4 cycles per second up to 8 cycles per second, Theta is present in dreaming sleep and provides the experience of deep meditation when you meditate. Theta also contains the storehouse of creative insp-iration and is where you often have your spiritual connection. Theta provides the "peak" in the peak experience.

Delta brainwaves are the unconscious mind, the deep sleep state, ranging from about 4 cycles per second down to 0.5 cycles per second. When present in combination with other waves in a waking state, Delta acts as a form of radar — seeking out information — reaching out to understand on the deepest unconscious level things that we can't understand through the thought process. Delta provides intuition, empathetic attunement, and instinctual insight. It is also the brain wave most often associated with energy healing.

Hemi-Sync® research has been ongoing for more than five decades, and today is concentrated in three distinct areas:

1. Clinical application by members of The Monroe Institute®'s Professional Division. This might involve, for example, studying Metamusic® as an aid for reducing anxiety in the dentist's waiting room.

2. Independent clinical research by universities or other institutions on the mechanisms underlying the effectiveness of the Hemi-Sync® process.

3. Applied research in The Monroe Institute® laboratory to imp-rove and expand Hemi-Sync® applications. The Institute uses

conventional scientific procedures whenever feasible but does not limit itself to such processes.

Learn more by visiting: https://hemi-sync.com/learn/research-papers.

A BIOGRAPHY OF ROBERT A. MONROE
(1915-1995)

Robert Monroe was a successful and distinguished business executive, dedicated family man, and noted pioneer in the investigation of human consciousness. He invented the Hemi-Sync® audio technology and founded The Monroe Institute®, a global organization dedicated to expanding the uses and understanding of consciousness.

Born in Indiana on October 30, 1915, to a college professor father and medical doctor mother, Robert Monroe was the third of four children. After a childhood spent in Kentucky and Indiana, he attended Ohio State University. Upon graduating in 1937 with a BA in English, Monroe worked as a writer and director at two Ohio radio stations. Two years later he moved to New York and expanded his broadcasting career, producing and directing weekly radio programs.

In 1953 Monroe formed RAM Enterprises, a corporation that produced network radio programs, as many as 28 programs monthly, principally in dramatic and popular quiz shows, including the popular *Take a Number* and *Meet Your Match* quiz shows. At this time Monroe became well known as a composer of music for radio, television, and motion pictures. He also served as vice president and a member of the board of directors for the Mutual Broadcasting System network, was listed in

Who's Who in America, and was publicized in magazine and newspaper articles on flying and radio production. Building on this success, Monroe's production company acquired several radio stations in North Carolina and Virginia and later moved into developing cable television systems.

In 1956 the firm set up a research and development division to study the effects of various sound patterns on human consciousness, including the feasibility of learning during sleep. Never one to ask others to do something he would not, Monroe often used himself as a test subject for this research. In 1958, a significant result emerged — Monroe began experiencing a state of consciousness separate and apart from the physical body. He described the state as an "out-of-body experience," the term popularized by Charles T. Tart, PhD. a leader in the area of consciousness studies. These spontaneous experiences altered the course of Monroe's life and the direction of his professional efforts.

In 1962 the company moved to Virginia, and a few years later changed the corporate name to Monroe Industries. In this location it became active in radio station ownership, cable television, and later in the production and sale of audio cassettes. These cassettes were practical expressions of the discoveries made in the earlier and ongoing corporate research program.

While continuing his successful broadcasting activities, Monroe began to experiment with and research the expanded forms of consciousness that he was experiencing. He chronicled his early explorations with a reporter's objectivity and eye for detail in a groundbreaking book, *Journeys Out of the Body*, which was published in 1971. This public record of his out-of-body experiences in states beyond space, time, and death has comforted countless people who've encountered paranormal incidents. It also attracted the attention of academic researchers, medical practitioners, engineers, and other professionals.

Ever the pragmatic business leader, Monroe and a growing group of fellow researchers began to work on methods of inducing and controlling this and other forms of consciousness in a laboratory setting. This research led to the development of a noninvasive and easy-to-use enhanced binaural beat audio guidance technology known as hemispheric synchronization, or Hemi-Sync®.

In 1974, the original research group was expanded to become The Monroe Institute of Applied Sciences, an organization dedicated to conducting seminars in the control and exploration of human consciousness. A year later, Monroe was issued the first of three patents for *Frequency Following Response* or FFR, which is part of the Hemi-Sync® method of altering brain states through sound.

Throughout the next 20 years Monroe continued to explore, research, and teach others about expanded states of human consciousness and practical methods of using them to enhance the experience of life. He developed a series of multi-day workshops that enable participants to personally access realms beyond physical time-space reality, built a campus for education and research, and created a portfolio of enhanced binaural beat audio exercises designed to focus attention, reduce stress, improve meditation, enhance sleep, and manage pain, among other applications.

In 1985 he wrote a second book, titled *Far Journeys*, which expanded upon his personal investigations of nonphysical reality. That same year the company officially changed its name, once again, to Interstate Industries, Inc. This reflected Monroe's analogy of how the use of Hemi-Sync® serves as a ramp from the "local road" to the "interstate" in allowing us to go full steam ahead in the exploration of con-sciousness, avoiding all of the stops and starts.

The research subsidiary was divested and established as an in-dependent non-profit organization, The Monroe Institute®, later in

1985. Interstate Industries, Inc. remains a privately-held company, now doing business as Hemi-Sync®.

In 1994 he followed suit with a third book, *Ultimate Journey*, which explores basic truths about the meaning and purpose of life and what lies beyond the limits of our physical world. Monroe died in 1995, at the age of 79. His legacy continues today and has touched the lives of literally millions of people all around the world.

RESOURCES FOR FURTHER WORK

This program will be beneficial for all those who need to improve their diet, lose excess weight, improve their activity levels and gain the many benefits of feeling healthier. The powerful messages in this program will support whatever improvements you wish to make.

DIABETICS

Type 1 diabetics must carefully balance blood sugar with medication, therefore the advice and support of your medical professional is essential before making any dietary changes.

Type 2 diabetics and those with pre-diabetes may benefit from losing weight. Consult your medical professional for advice. The American Diabetes Association website is a useful resource of information about healthy eating, in particular reducing carbohydrate consumption. Visit https://www.diabetes.org

OTHER DIETARY LIMITATIONS

It is not uncommon for people to limit certain foods because they "do not love you back." Certain foods or food groups may make you feel unwell or be harmful to you. There may be moral or religious reasons for excluding certain foods. Plant-based diets are growing in popularity. You can include all these dietary limitations within this program. As you listen carefully to what your body tells you as you progress, you will gain useful insights about ensuring you eat foods that nourish every part of you so you can create your slim, healthy body and enhance your wellbeing.

ACUTAPPING
Track 4 introduces a specially designed acutapping procedure that will "dissolve the threads that bind you" to your craving foods. Track 10 continues with a modified acutapping procedure to reverse the behavior of self-sabotage. However, acutapping has many other benefits and you may wish to explore this complementary therapy further.

Acutapping is a collective term to describe the process of combining the manual stimulation of certain acupuncture points while focusing on an emotional, psychological or physical issue, and by doing so, gain healing and resolution. Many innovative professionals in the field of conventional and complementary medicine have contributed to the discovery and advancement of this work. Acutapping is available in many forms, and it is not possible to list each of the variations that are available worldwide.

A useful starting point is the book by Dr. Roger Callahan — *Tapping the Healer Within* — (McGraw-Hill Education, January 2001) which des-cribes Thought Field Therapy (TFT).

There are many books to purchase by many of the pioneers that can provide a background to this growing field of complementary therapy.

Gary Craig is one such innovator who simplified and reconfigured the acutapping process into Emotional Freedom Technique (EFT) which is designed to be self-applied once the procedure has been learned. EFT was promoted worldwide via the internet and those early EFT pioneers who spread the word. More information, articles, free resources and practitioner listings are available by visiting Gary Craig's website: https://www.emofree.com.

EFT International is an organization which brings together EFT practitioners worldwide. Their website states: "EFT International is committed to advancing and upholding the highest standards for education, training, professional development and promotion of the skilful, creative and ethical application of EFT." You can find information, free resources and a directory of accredited EFT practitioners by visiting https://www.eftinternational.org.

Other acutapping therapies or energy therapies include:

- Be Set Free Fast
- Emotrance
- The Choices Method in EFT
- Freeway CER

If you choose to work one-to-one with a therapist, ensure your chosen therapist is well qualified, experienced and a member of a suitable professional body. Effective therapy requires trust and cooperation, therefore it makes sense to work with a therapist you feel comfortable with.

I am indebted to Jenny McCarthy, shiatsu practitioner and Reiki Master for help with designing the craving control procedure. *Ocean of Steams — Shiatsu Meridians, Tsubos and Theoretical Impressions* by Veet John Allan MRSS, provided valuable background information.

HYPNOTHERAPY
If you feel you would benefit from individual sessions with a therapist, I hope this program will give you the insight and confidence to work on those aspects of your weight loss journey that may need a targeted

approach. Everything you experience in these 12 guided meditations will support you in any one-to-one work you choose to do. You will already have the basics covered and this will greatly assist you if you decide to work with a therapist on aspects of your weight loss that require ongoing personal support.

There are different accreditation requirements for different countries. In some places, hypnotherapists must also be medically qualified, whereas in others it is a complementary therapy. However, all such therapists have to be trained to a high standard, belong to a suitable professional body and be registered to practice by the appropriate authority.

Choose a therapist who you feel comfortable with, who is a specialist in this subject and who is open to complementing your work with this album of guided meditations.

The website:
www.slimmerandhealthierforlife.com
offers further advice, support and a regular blog so you can keep in touch as you progress on your journey.

Alternatively, visit Deborah's hypnotherapy website at:
www.db-hypnosis.co.uk
and follow the link to the *Slimmer and Healthier* dedicated website.

ACKNOWLEDGMENTS

With sincere appreciation to all at Hemi-Sync® for all the hard work, enthusiasm and energy that has gone into the creation of this 12 track album and companion book.

I am indebted to Carol Moore for having confidence in this product and for her continued support. Carol's contribution of Robert Monroe's biography is a welcome addition to this book, allowing readers who are not familiar with the back story of Hemi-Sync® to gain a deeper understanding.

Many thanks are due to Hemi-Sync® Chairman and President Garrett Stevens for understanding the possibilities of publishing a companion book and extending the support to make it happen.

Judy Madison has guided me through the editing process. I am very grateful for her insights, eye for detail, patience and expertise.

Kevin Cowan and his team are to be congratulated for the inspiring sound engineering work that brings the guided meditations to life. Christopher Lloyd Clarke's music perfects the final product.

Dan Marshall of In-Phase Studios, Bedfordshire, UK, deserves great credit for the voice recording process and the fun we had while turning the 12 scripts into audio tracks.

Kelly-Marie Parker of Kel's Belles salon in Bedford, UK, modeled and photographed the acutapping points for me.

Jenny McCarthy, Shiatsu practitioner and Reiki Master, provided valuable support and expertise when I was designing the unique acutapping procedure for Tracks 4 and 9.

Finally, there are many individuals over the last 20 years who have entrusted me with their own personal journeys towards a slim, healthy body. Their insights and experiences have honed and shaped this process, providing me with the necessary depth of understanding to create this 12 track program and companion book.

My intention has always been to make losing weight and creating a slim, healthy body an enjoyable and positive experience. By doing so, success is easily achievable. I sincerely hope that all who struggle with their weight will find their slim, healthy self by following this program and go on to get the most out of this wonderful life.

CPSIA information can be obtained
at www.ICGtesting.com
Printed in the USA
LVHW030811240320
651022LV00013B/2659